Liposuction and Plastic Surgery of the Abdomen

For Churchill Livingstone:
Publisher: Georgina Bentliff
Project Editor: Lucy Gardner
Copy Editor: Jennifer Bew
Indexer: Helen McKillop
Production Controller: Nancy Henry
Sales Promotion Executive: Louise Johnstone

Liposuction and Plastic Surgery of the Abdomen

J. S. Elbaz MD

Vice Président du Club des Professeurs et Professionnels de Chirurgie Plastique et Esthétique; Secrétaire Général du Collège Français d'Enseignement de Chirurgie Plastique et Esthétique; Ancien Président de la Société Française de Chirurgie Plastique Reconstructrice et Esthétique; Secrétaire Général du Chapitre de Chirurgie Esthétique de la Société Française de Chirurgie Plastique et Esthétique; Expert National près de la Cour de Cassation; Expert Clinicien auprès du Ministère de la Santé; Membre de l'International Society of Plastic Reconstructive Surgery; Membre de l'International Society of Aesthetic Plastic Surgery

G. Flageul MD

Chirurgien des Hôpitaux de Paris

With the collaboration of
J. C. Dardour, V. Mitz, S. H. Abraham and **E. Sitbon**

Translated by
Charles-Henri Caillile MD

CHURCHILL LIVINGSTONE
EDINBURGH LONDON MADRID MELBOURNE NEW YORK AND TOKYO 1993

CHURCHILL LIVINGSTONE
Medical Division of Longman Group UK Limited

Distributed in the United States of America by Churchill
Livingstone Inc., 650 Avenue of the Americas, New York,
N.Y. 10011, and by associated companies, branches and
representatives throughout the world.

English translation © Longman Group UK Limited 1993

Liposuccion et Chirurgie Plastique de L'Abdomen 2E,
J. S. Elbaz & G. Flageul
© Masson, Editeur, Paris, 1989

First English edition 1993

ISBN 0-443-04637-9

British Library of Cataloguing in Publication Data
A catalogue record for this book is available from the
British Library.

Library of Congress Cataloging in Publication Data
Elbaz, J. S. (Jean-Sauveur)
     [Liposuccion et chirurgie plastique de l'abdomen.
     English]
     Liposuction and plastic surgery of the abdomen / Jean
     Sauveur
Elbaz, Gerard Flageul; with the collaboration of
J. C. Dardour . . . [et al.]; translated by
Charles-Henri Caillile.
          p.   cm.
     Translation of: Liposuccion et chirurgie plastique de
     l'abdomen.
     Includes index.
     1. Abdomen — Surgery. 2. Surgery, Plastic.
     3. Liposuction.
     I. Flageul. G. (Gérard) II. Title.
     [DNLM: 1. Abdomen — surgery. 2. Lipectomy.
     3. Surgery, Plastic.
     WI 900 W37L]
     RD119.5.A24E4313   1992
     617.5′50592 — dc20
     DNLM/DLC
     for Library of Congress   92–15510
                                                CIP

Produced by Longman Singapore Publishers Pte Ltd
Printed in Singapore

Contents

1. Historical introduction

In the first (1977) edition of this book we explained that these operations were being performed more and more often because of a largely psychological demand; for a woman, the abdomen is a potent symbol of her femininity.

These cosmetic operations, unquestionably stemming from general surgery, seemed to us at the time to have been little studied, and from the start we emphasized the importance of scarring, which no method seemed to have taken into consideration. As we said then, without discussing the fundamental differences in culture which accept or reject the exposure of the female body, we must remember that western civilizations are tending to strip more and more often, and it is attempting the impossible to try to hide a scar under female underwear. This is why in 1974 we proposed a low and localized incision, without umbilical transposition leaving a minimal scar.

Among the different clinical pictures, we distinguished the following:

- The obese patient
- The patient with abdominal scars
- Distended and stretchmarked abdomens
- Dermal dystrophies

It is an undoubted fact that even one pregnancy can damage the abdomen of a woman: statistically this is quite evident.

Many primiparous and multiparous women go through pregnancy unharmed; this is good, but other women are affected by the mechanical factor of distension of the abdominal wall, by hormonal flooding, by tissue modifications and by general weight gain. This is an obvious clinical reality.

Is there then such a thing as aesthetic damage due to pregnancy? Reservedly, yes; thanks to contraception, voluntary pregnancy is evidently more than desirable, but western women no longer wish to suffer its 'damage'. We must also ask ourselves if the cost of correcting this 'aesthetic damage' should be borne by the social services, originally set up for serious ailments and representing nationally a very heavy economic burden.

Technical progress in abdominal plastic surgery over the last 25 years has been considerable. Let us summarize the major stages.

THE FIRST OPERATIONS

In 1959, Dufourmentel and Mouly described a low transverse dermo-lipectomy procedure with an umbilical transposition that became classic. In 1960, Mario González Ulloa described a circular dermo-lipectomy later taken up by Vilain in France. In 1967, Pitanguy on the one hand and Callia on the other described their original techniques. All these procedures had three points in common:

1. They all involved umbilical transposition — in fact a pseudotransposition, since the umbilicus remained in its place.
2. The supraumbilical point had to become suprapubic at all costs, regardless of the state of the abdomen (obese, wrinkled, stretchmarked or scarred), and regardless of the general shape of the abdomen. This prevented all surgical treatment for moderate abdominal lesions.
3. The result was a very long and very prominent low transverse scar, which unfortunately is often much higher on

1

postoperative pictures than in the sketches in the medical literature. The distance between the umbilicus and the pubic triangle that we have described as about 13 cm is often very short. Finally, it is not uncommon to observe a deformation of the pubic triangle due to spreading or ascension.

In short, in these important low transverse abdominoplasties with umbilical transposition, even if the patient was psychologically happy with the result, the cosmetic aspect missed the point: the surgery was performed more to permit dressing than undressing. Certain humorists described these abdominoplasties as 'abominoplasties', that plastic surgeons detested performing.

DEFINITIVE CONTRIBUTIONS

Since 1974, we have promoted a low and localized abdominoplasty intended for moderate and essentially subumbilical lesions. This is known as the horseshoe technique (Elbaz 1974). Three main ideas guided this kind of operation:

1. To reduce as much as possible the length of the scar, and preferably conceal it totally in the pubic triangle.
2. If requested, to place the fatty cutaneous subumbilical layer of the abdomen under normal tension, exactly as in face lifting.
3. To drop the 'compulsory figure', as we say in ice skating, that is, the umbilical transposition.

The umbilicus, right in the middle of the abdomen, was holding us back.

We summed up our points of view about these operations in *Plastic Surgery of the Abdomen*, published in France in 1977; subsequently in the United States in 1979.

Since the problem of the scar has become the main concern for many surgeons, publications concerning the techniques of adapting cutaneous resection to the lesion have increased markedly.

The second main contribution was the arrival in 1978 of atraumatic liposuction by the wet tunnels method of Illouz; this respects the arteriovenous vascularization and avoids the cre-

ation of a single cavity. It is now recognized that isolated liposuction of the abdomen can give excellent results. The abdomen, however, is one of the most difficult and unforgiving areas, given the residual asymmetry and the difficulty sometimes of appraising the strength of skin retraction in the preoperative stage. In cases of foreseeable excess of skin, cutaneous reduction surgery will be automatically performed.

The third contribution was to restore the use of umbilical disinsertion, described by Callia as early as 1965; easy to carry out with a low transverse approach, it allows the umbilicus to be moved down by 2–3 cm, and the fatty-cutaneous layers of the abdomen above and below the umbilicus to be put under normal tension. At the same time it respects a proper umbilicus–pubic triangle distance (11 cm minimum).

The fourth important contribution seems to us to be the sophisticated technique intended to put under tension the musculo–aponeurotic layer when this has been distended.

Finally, the last technical contribution is the use of 'fibrin glue' consisting of fibrinogen and thrombin. When put together by spraying, these two products lead to the formation of fibrin, a true 'glue' that realizes the last stage of blood coagulation. Its advantages are:

1. It eliminates detachment in 2 minutes.
2. It reinforces haemostasis, but this should obviously remain meticulous.
3. It possibly ensures lymphostasis, considerably diminishing the appearance of seroma or Morel–Lavallée discharge.
4. It eliminates drainage.
5. It diminishes traction on the suture.

Thus, after a long development it seems that abdominal plastic surgery has become a genuinely cosmetic operation. For moderate abdominal lesions, we propose a low and localized abdominoplasty or ASA (aesthetic suction abdominoplasty) consisting of primary liposuction with or without umbilical disinsertion; the use of a fibrin glue; a horseshoe incision which is practically concealed by the pubic triangle. In this way, we are beginning to see some very satisfactory results with abdominoplasty.

2. The abdominal wall and anatomy of the figure

According to the definition of Littré, the figure is 'a projected shadow forming a shape'. We cannot discuss mammoplasty, correction of the thighs and trochanteric areas, and especially abdominoplasty, without studying the various parts of the body in relation to its entirety, with the patient in the upright or anatomical position.

Morphology deals with the external form of the body or its fatty-cutaneous covering, as opposed to anatomy, which is the study of its internal structures. The study of morphology is a necessity for the plastic surgeon, who, due to his classical surgical training, often limits his knowledge to the anatomical elements. However, morphology has been carefully studied in its clinical aspects, its variations (biotyping or anthropometry) and their relationship to sex, growth, or ageing.

WHAT ARE THE FACTORS DETERMINING MORPHOLOGY?

The shape of the body is the result of three fundamental elements: (1) a bony framework, covered by (2) red striated muscle, which itself is covered by (3) a fatty-cutaneous envelope. These three elements depend on a certain number of secondary factors, such as heredity, endocrine factors and eating habits (Fig. 2.1).

As to the bony structure, the only difference between a man and a woman is in the pelvis, owing to the role of the female pelvis in childbirth. Women have a wider pelvis which is not as high as a man's, and the inferior opening is larger.

Concerning the musculature, the strap muscles of the female are identical to those of the male, except that they are generally smaller, yet there are some athletic women whose muscles are often

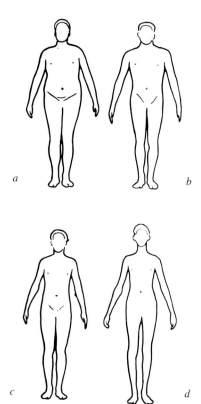

Fig. 2.1 Sheldon's types: **a** endomorph; **b** mesomorph; **c** average type; **d** ectomorph.

more developed than those of the average man.

The main difference between male and female morphology can be found in the distribution of body fat. Fat is located in two main parts of the human body with regard to the general musculo-aponeurosis:

Subaponeurotic: this accumulates in the area of the muscular interstices, i.e. along the neurovascular channels; this is interstitial adipose tissue.

3

Supraaponeurotic: this is the major type of fat. It is located directly beneath the skin and is closely adherent to it. It constitutes the 'panniculus adiposus', more or less equally distributed, which cushions the muscular and bony angles. This subcutaneous adipose panniculus (SAP) is measured with a caliper, which gives two thicknesses of skin and two of fat. We can analyse this panniculus with two complementary studies: xerography and echography.

Fat has a major impact on the morphology, whether it be hypertrophied or atrophied, generalized or localized. The most eloquent clinical manifestation of fat distribution is seen in the Barraquers–Simmons syndrome.

The locations of this SAP are not the same for the two sexes, and variations give the true difference, as far as the figure is concerned, between men and women.

ANATOMICAL ELEMENTS OF THE ABDOMINAL STRUCTURE

After an analytical approach, the four elements contributing to the shape of the abdomen will be described: the skeleton, muscles, subcutaneous fat and skin. The umbilicus will be studied separately because of its surgical importance.

Skeleton

The skeleton is composed of the posterior, superior, and inferior sections. **The posterior section** is . made up of the spine, with its physiological kyphosis and the lumbar lordosis. Any deformity in this segment will cause a change in the shape of the abdomen, which is temporarily evident in the case of pregnant women. Any accentuation of the lordosis, especially in the case of certain black people, will lead to a forward projection of the abdominal wall, which is convex in front. It would be desirable to complete the clinical study with a profile of the lumbar area of the back.

The upper section corresponds to the lower opening of the thorax, marked from back to front by the lower rim of the tenth rib, the last six costal cartilages, and the xiphoid process. It is obvious that the anterior portion of this thoracic opening with a somewhat accentuated frontal curve will determine the shape of the abdominal muscles.

The lower section is simply the upper approach of the pelvis. From back to front it includes the promontory, the anterior border of the sacral wing, the innominate line, and the superior border of the symphysis pubis.

It has already been pointed out that women have a wider and lower pelvis than men; their iliac bones are more flared and they project further to the outside; the lower opening is wider; the pubic symphysis is lower; the concavity of the sacrococcygeal angle is more pronounced; and the ischial tuberosities are further apart from each other. Richer has devised a mean statistic shown in Table 2.1.

Table 2.1

	M	F
Biiliac diameter (cm)	28	30
Height (cm)	20	18

We must conclude from the shape of the bone structure that any deformity of the spine will influence the shape of the abdominal profile. This is evident in the case of accentuated lumbar lordosis, which causes forward projection of the abdominal wall, a physiological trait in certain populations, such as black people. It would be unreasonable to promise such people a flat abdomen, since surgery would not be able to accomplish this. We must stress the importance of a careful preoperative radiographic examination for such bony abnormalities (Fig. 2.2).

Muscles

The classic pattern of the three large muscles of the anterolateral region of the abdominal wall, namely, the external oblique, the internal oblique, and the transversus, which ends at the outside end of the rectus abdominis, will not be emphasized.

The fact that the shape of the white line is different in its upper two-thirds from its lower

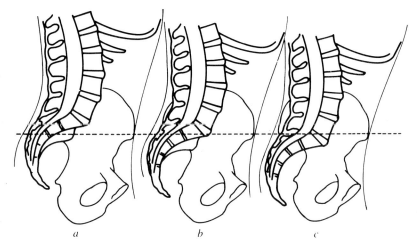

Fig. 2.2 Position of the sacrum in relation to the pelvis. **a** Normal position; **b** sacrum in a high position; **c** sacrum embedded in the pelvis — as a result, in the three cases, the height of the thigh is different, as one can see on these diagrams from the interval separating the last rib from the iliac crest. The horizontal dotted line runs through the three figures at the same level of the hip bone.

third is well known. Suffice it to say that a diastasis recti cannot be considered unless the space between the inner borders of the muscles is greater than 4 cm. This anterolateral wall of the abdomen, which is stretched between the opening of the rib cage at the top and the iliac basin at the bottom, appears as a segment of the musculoaponeurotic cylinder supported in the back by the articulations of the spine and its paravertebral muscles cords. Four practical conclusions can be drawn from this spatial geometric structure:

1. The transverse curve of this area is determined by the upper and lower borders; therefore the flatter the costal opening, the flatter the abdomen.
2. The quality of the muscles and aponeurosis of the abdomen is determined by the 'thrust' of the abdominal organs, which is referred to as 'turgor'. This thrust is contained by the diaphragm in the upper part, the pelvic floor at the base, and the abdominal wall in front. It is difficult to maintain this abdominal turgor in its entirety, especially in cases of obesity or pregnancy, and even more so at its anatomical weak points, such as the white line, the umbilicus, and the inguinal canal and ring.

3. It is obvious that good abdominal musculature and the development of these muscles is important for the general state of the abdomen.
4. Finally, surgically created abdominal scars add to the weakness of the overall abdominal wall.

Subcutaneous fat

Unfortunately, anatomists disregard fat and start their study of the human body with the muscles and the skeleton. Nor has adipose tissue ever been adequately studied by surgeons, to whom it has always been a great cause for concern. Adipose tissue is a connective tissue composed of round fat cells whose diameter varies between 50 and 150 μ, each containing a large fat globule. This adipose tissue is very abundant in the abdominal wall, which is the third largest area of fat deposit in the body (the largest areas are the buttocks and the bulge over the hips). In the obese patient, there is more fat in the abdominal wall than anywhere else in the body.

In women, this fat accumulates mainly in the periumbilical region and between the waist and the inferior abdominal fold (Fig. 2.3). The defi-

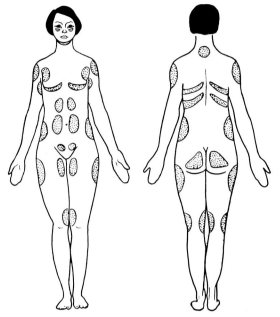

Fig. 2.3 The main areas of fat deposition in a female.

nition of the major abdominal muscles, which are very visible in a well-developed male, is less obvious in the female due to this subcutaneous periumbilical fat. Any degree of weight gain in

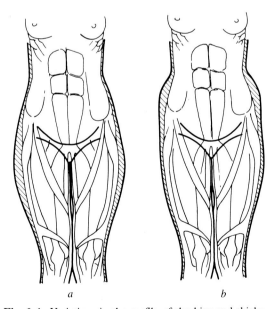

Fig. 2.4 Variations in the profile of the hips and thighs according to the degree of subtrochanteric fat deposition **a** or on the hips **b** In both figures the musculoskeletal silhouette is the same.

the abdominal area in a woman will result in a round stomach, both frontally and laterally, and there will be a greater amount of fat below the navel. **In the male** the reverse is true: the fat tends to accumulate over the navel.

In both sexes, excess abdominal fat tends to be deposited laterally in a bulge over the hips, marked on either side by the upper and lower lumbar sulci, and evident in the anatomical position, stopping just a few centimetres over the line of the lower ribs (Fig. 2.4).

Fat, therefore, is at the root of the abdomen's morphology, giving the belly a rounded shape. The quantity of fat stocked at this level varies greatly, hence the variety of abdominal morphologies.

Two distinct layers of fat should be distinguished, superficial and deep.

Superficial or areolar fat

At the abdominal level, the fat is found above the fascia superficialis. Only small vessels run through it to supply the skin. This superficial fat is what is involved in cellulite and its effect on the skin, particularly the 'orange peel' appearance is due to the aponeurotic fixation tracts reaching the deep side of the skin. Its thickness is well known and varies very little for a determined area. For the abdominal wall, the average thickness is between 0.8 and 1.2 cm for a thin person, and between 1.4 and 2 cm for a fat one.

Liposuction will nor be concerned with this type of fat because it is superficial; it corresponds to a 'safety thickness' beneath which the cannula should pass, so as not to leave a mark.

Deep reticular or lamellar fat

This is situated directly beneath the superficial fat, from which it is separated at the abdominal wall level by the fascia superficialis. This is where the largest blood and lymphatic vessels that supply the skin are situated. This deep layer could be the site of localized excess fat deposits, that deform the figure.

The term 'lipodistrophy' in this case is not valid because this excess fat buildup is neither pathological nor dystrophic; rather the term 'fat deposit' seems more suitable, since it is semantically logical, disregards any pathology and insists on the localized character of this fatty formation. Fat deposits are normal heaps of fat in locations determined by a genetic code.

Contrary to certain opinions, it seems that the deep fat is the one more likely to hypertrophy in cases of a general excess of weight. Thus at the abdominal wall level, this deep layer (0.5 cm in a thin subject) reaches a thickness of 3.2–4.5 cm in a fat subject. In this case, the superficial fascia, which is subdivided into 4–10 layers, undergoes a substantial increase in thickness.

This deep fat will be the one essentially involved in liposuction. Xerography and echography allow us to appreciate and objectivize this adipose envelope.

The most important fat deposits are those on the eyelids, chin, hips, thighs, knees, leg, abdomen and the supramammary region. It seems that there is a difference in the composition of the fatty tissue between the subumbilical and the supraumbilical fat. The fat deposits on the hips and abdomen will determine the morphology of the abdominal wall and the belly in general.

Abdominal fat deposit

A flat belly is the result of very little fat deposit. The increase in this fat deposit determines the classic aspects of the 'small tummy' or the 'large tummy'. It should be noted that the fat above the superficial fascia affects the whole abdominal wall; as for the deep fat beneath the superficial fascia, this is essentially subumbilical and lateroumbilical.

Hips fat deposit

At this level, we should distinguish the fat deposit that forms a roll of fat (the lateral roll of the sides), and could become what is commonly known as a 'spare tyre', from the fat deposit that corresponds to the classic 'riding breeches'. This does not concern us here.

Skin

Abdominal skin is quite thick when compared with skin in other parts of the body (2–4 mm). It is very elastic, with a rich blood supply, and stretches easily in the case of pregnancy and obesity. Its elasticity is limited, however, when it comes to regaining its original shape once the cause of distension has been removed. The elasticity then is dependent on the degree of distension, endocrine factors, and the age of the patient.

The appraisal of elasticity is an essential preoperative element of surgery and therapeutic strategy. Its importance is increased by the effects of liposuction; we know that following liposuction we should 'drape' the skin over the new contours in order to adapt the 'container' to the 'new contents'; this redraping happens by itself if the skin has remained sufficiently elastic. On the other hand, if that spontaneous redraping is insufficient, a skin reduction plasty should be carried out. This will leave a prominent scar.

This is one reason why it is very important to be able to judge the necessity or otherwise for skin reduction plasty before surgery. This requires the ability to evaluate the spontaneous redraping capability of the skin, and that depends on its biomechanical qualities. These are very variable from one patient to another and are not easily assessed with precision. Clinical experience plays an important part here, together with the assessment of various parameters and different tests, which will be studied in Chapter 7, dealing with the mechanical properties of the abdominal wall. They will be briefly mentioned here:

1. The relation between the volume of aspirated fat and the area of skin involved.
2. The legal age.
3. Physiological cutaneous age: thickness, extensibility, signs of local premature ageing (stretchmarks).
4. The abdominal localization: this is not the most favourable region, unlike the riding breeches, the knee and the region under the chin, for example. Abdominal liposuction is nevertheless frequently useful, but one should be careful in this appraisal of the ability of the skin to redrape spontaneously, principally

when an isolated abdominal liposuction without skin reduction plasty is considered. This is because the skin of the abdominal wall does not have the highest retraction power, as it could have been distended prematurely and aged by pregnancy or an alternating sequence of weight gain and loss. It is here that the tests are useful.

5. The tests: pinch test; compression test; Illouz's muscular inspection test.

We must now see the relationship between the pubic triangle and the body landmarks. The pubic triangle is found over the anterior part of the pubis, which connects laterally to the ischio-pubic and iliopubic rami, and medially to the pubic symphysis. The upper part of the triangle, traditionally straight in the female, extends over the edge of the pubic bone by 2–3 cm. Note that its border remains separate from the lower abdominal fold with the concavity of the arc going upward, between the two anterior superior iliac spines, marking the lower pole of the abdomen.

Anatomically the anterior portion of the female genitalia is fixed to its bony support by the labia, the corpus cavernosus, and the clitoris. This degree of anatomical fixation (mobility) depends on the amount of fat surrounding the round ligaments and the mons pubis. It is important to consider the relationship between the pubic triangle and the underlying structures when performing an abdominoplasty, to avoid the undesirable consequence of advancing the pubic triangle too far upwards.

The distance between the umbilicus and the upper border of the pubic triangle was studied on 100 women with so-called normal abdomens, and found to be remarkably constant — approximately 13 cm, regardless of the weight or size of the patient (Fig. 2.5).

THE UMBILICUS

This must be studied separately, since it is very important both from an anatomical and a surgical point of view. The umbilical morphology, its topography and finally its situation will be considered.

Morphology

The umbilicus is not superficial, but is always situated at the bottom of a crater whose depth depends on the abundance of the surrounding fat. Regardless of the degree of obesity it will never flatten out, and its exteriorization during abdominoplasties should take into account this anatomical configuration.

Apart from its universally recognized 'hole-shaped' characteristic, the other morphological parameters of the umbilicus appear very variable. Beside the classic round umbilicus we find the umbilicus with a large vertical or horizontal axis, the half-moon umbilicus, the button-shaped umbilicus, the 'coffee-bean' umbilicus, the 'cat's eye' umbilicus, the asymmetrical umbilicus, and so on. In addition to these anatomical curiosities, it seems that its roundness and its depth are the two most vividly described aesthetic virtues.

Topography and situation (Figs. 2.6, 2.7)

The umbilicus usually projects at the intersection of the midpoint of a vertical line and a horizontal transverse line, at the highest point of the iliac crests; this is a classic notion that was confirmed by the work of Dubou and Ousterhout (1978) based on 100 patients. This places it at an

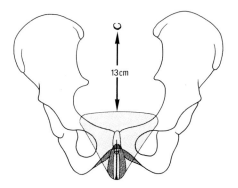

Fig. 2.5 Forward projection of the vulva on the skeleton. The gray triangle represents the pubic hair. It is usually an equilateral triangle, measuring 10 cms on each side. The lower angle of the triangle is bounded by the bulbocavernosis and ischiocavernosis muscles. When the tension is placed on the lower portion of the abdomen, the escutcheon will advance upward, relative to the degree of elasticity.

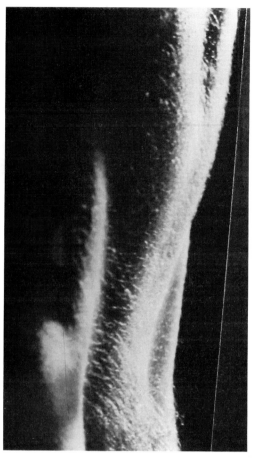

Fig. 2.6 Umbilicus in position in the rectus abdominus muscle. Here, the predominant axis is longitudinal.

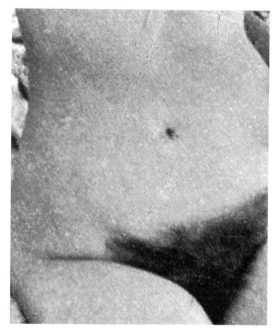

Fig. 2.7 Patient with a small, round umbilicus. There is an abundant amount of hair considering a 13 cm umbilico-pubic distance.

average distance of 6 cm above the anterosuperior iliac spines.

The projection of the umbilicus on the spinal column corresponds to the intervertebral disc situated between the third and fourth lumbar vertebrae. Finally, note that the umbilicus is situated approximately halfway between the xiphoid and the pubis, as has been confirmed by the above mentioned work (Dubou & Ousterhout 1978).

In conclusion, when considering the abdomen in relation to the rest of the anatomy, the following should be taken into account.

- Biiliac diameter
- Biacromial diameter
- Chest, waist and hip measurements

- Distance between umbilicus and pubis, which strangely enough is constant in most women, i.e. 13 cm,
- Thickness of the skin fold
- Weight of the subject
- Height of the subject

Even the clothing industry manufactures garments with these constant measurements in mind. During our study, we have used a diagram to chart our results.

To conclude, one fact remains clear: there is a great difference between long and wide abdomens, considering the skeleton, muscles and fat, as well as the ratio between the biiliac diameter and umbilicopubic distance. When planning an operation, the most important measurement to consider is the distance between the sternum and the pubis. Since the abdominal flap is pulled down toward the pubis and amputated, it will be necessary to recreate a normal relative distance between the xiphoid–umbilicus and the umbilicus–pubis in order to assure proper placement of the umbilicus. In other words, the wide abdomen has a biiliac diameter which is large compared to the umbilicopubic distance. After resection of the abdominal flap, it will be easier to approximate the skin edges and to correct the 'dog ears'.

On the other hand, in a long abdomen the biiliac diameter is less in relation to the umbilico-pubic distance. In this case, it will be more difficult to approximate the abdominal flap to the pubis. This problem is always encountered in plastic surgery when a circle must be stitched.

Between these two extremes lie many intermediary shapes. This distinction, while it may seem general, is very important to consider when planning an operation. It will be referred to again.

3. The various clinical pictures

For the sake of simplicity, consider three separate groups of patients, each requiring abdominal correction for a different reason, although sometimes more than one condition may be seen in the same patient:

1. The obese patient.
2. Patients who have abdominal scars, both surgical and traumatic.
3. Patients with distended abdomens, often the aesthetic price paid for one or many pregnancies (these include pendulous wrinkled skin, as well as striae or stretchmarks).

Two different surgical rationales can be considered: for the obese person, operation is often indicated after consultation with the internist and surgeon, and the results will be impressive, with rapid diminution of the panniculus, although often the scars are less than aesthetically pleasing. On the other hand, patients with scarred abdomens, as well as those with wrinkled, stretched and pendulous skin, can have a more elective type of procedure, with somewhat better results.

THE OBESE PATIENT (Fig. 3.1)

Obese individuals constitute the majority of patients, both male and female, who require abdominal lipectomy. Liposuction has radically modified the surgical approach to such patients, however, since obesity is not in itself a disease but the common symptom of many different diseases, the patients who fall into this category differ greatly. Considerations are the patient's body type, degree of obesity, age, willingness to continue the postoperative medical treatment, and emotional status with regard to body image.

First, take the case of the truly obese patient who is either not willing or not able to reduce his weight. Here a possible solution would be the surgical excision of excess abdominal fat, which would solve his problems once and for all. The lipectomies, the so-called primary solution to the problem, are to be avoided at all costs. Certainly,

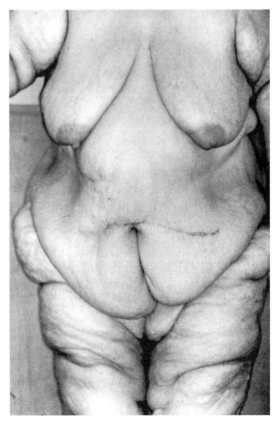

Fig. 3.1 Pendulous abdomen and excess abdominal fat in obese patient.

11

surgical intervention will remove fat and cause a layer of fibrous tissue to form in the area, which will deter future fatty deposits from forming, but it will never replace the willpower of the patient to follow a regulated sensible diet, or to investigate the problems of heredity or metabolism which may apply to his case.

This is where liposuction could help, but these patients should be referred to a weight reduction clinic, put on a low-calorie diet (without the use of dangerous drugs such as thyroid extract or diuretics), or put under psychiatric care to lose their excess weight.

An obese patient who has lost weight with the help of psychotherapy is clearly the ideal case. Depending on the age of the patient and the degree of elasticity of his skin, if there has been a significant weight loss (15–50 kg or more) the loss of subcutaneous fat usually brings about a ptosis of the skin (with an increase in the distance from the umbilicus to the pubic triangle), resulting in an abdominal apron or pendulous abdomen. This is quite noticeable when the patient is standing upright, and becomes worse when he leans forward. It can be measured by the distance between the umbilicus and the pubic triangle and constitutes an obvious physical deformity. Psychologically it changes the patient's body image; functionally it is uncomfortable and embarrassing, and pathologically it causes intertrigo and microclimates in the folds of the skin. Moreover, it presents clearcut risks in the event of surgical intervention for laparotomy. It is in these cases that the so-called secondary abdominoplasty is indicated.

Most physicians agree that after a significant weight loss, those truly obese patients who want to lose more weight could benefit from surgery, inasmuch as an alteration in their body image can give them a psychological impetus to adhere to their diet. In fact, very rarely do patients regain weight after this surgery, since a continued weight-loss programme is often carried out during a long hospitalization. If weight is regained after liposuction, it is done harmoniously.

The third group of obese patients consists of those who, in spite of a special diet within a controlled environment, and with all the usual psychological adjuncts, cannot lose any weight:

the adipose tissue of the abdomen is immobile. In these cases, abdominal lipectomy can benefit the patient by decreasing the amount of adipose tissue present. In these cases also, there should be a conference including the internist, surgeon, psychologist and patient.

PATIENTS WITH TRAUMATIC OR SURGICAL ABDOMINAL SCARS

All surgeons have seen patients with scars from appendectomy, peritonitis, caesarean section or cholecystectomy (Fig. 3.2). Also seen are scars due to the repair of umbilical hernia, eventration, and even evisceration. It is certainly reasonable, if there are no contraindications, to attempt to remove, if possible, part or all of these scars with abdominal reconstruction.

In other cases, the musculoaponeurotic wall has no surgical trauma, and the damage is limited to one or more bad scars (Fig. 3.3). The surgeon may be faced with a dehiscent scar that had healed by secondary intention, a midline hypertrophic scar, a keloid, or an adhesion deep into the fascial level, separating the fat and causing it to bunch at the muscular layer, and giving the appearance of a buttock-like' belly when standing, or the impression of 'rosary beads' when

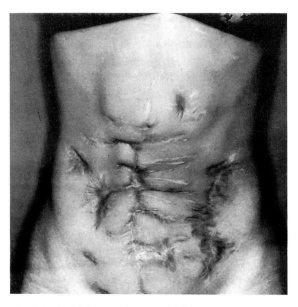

Fig. 3.2 Multiple scars from peritonitis.

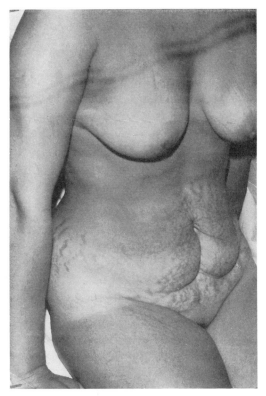

Fig. 3.3 Distended and stretch marked abdominal wall.

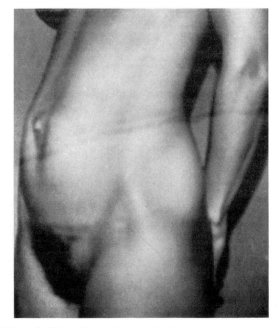

Fig. 3.4 Distended abdomen with diastasis recti.

sitting. Whatever the case may be, abdominoplasty will attempt to remove the adhesions, reconstruct the subcutaneous fat, and place proper tension on the overlying skin. Such an operation is indicated only for cosmetic improvement.

THE DISTENDED ABDOMEN

These cases are almost exclusively young and energetic women, with or without justification for changing their personal body image. The skin of the abdomen is wrinkled, creased, and has transverse pleats when the patient is sitting that become worse as she leans forward. Frequently there are associated stretchmarks, and it is important to take note of their colour, direction, size, location, and increase or decrease in severity (Fig. 3.4). The cause of these lesions is almost always pregnancy, although alternating periods of weight loss and weight gain, which can be learned from a careful history, seem to have a certain role as well.

In those cases where the patient seeks a purely cosmetic operation, the physician must carefully examine her motivations for having surgery. The plastic surgeon must explain the principles of the surgery, stress its limitations and the impossibility of total reconstruction, and must demonstrate the shape and length of the resulting scars. He should warn the patient that it may take months before the scars become 'acceptable'. Thus, by selecting the patient carefully, the surgeon will obtain the best possible results from both the physical and the psychological points of view, and will avoid as far as possible the dissatisfied patient.

Next to obesity and weight-loss programs, which are more or less successful, pregnancy seems to be one of the major indications for abdominoplasty, and deserves special mention with regard to the physiological changes seen in the abdominal wall. Most general practitioners and gynaecologists feel that a woman's body is not greatly changed during the various stages of pregnancy; however, the plastic surgeon, who sees women whose bodies *have* been deformed by pregnancy, may disagree with this thinking. This apparent contradiction highlights the disparity between different women. There is clinical evidence to show that certain women could carry several pregnancies without these leaving any disfiguring mark on the body. Some even find that pregnancy causes them to 'bloom'. Others, on the contrary, suffer disfiguring changes from the first months of pregnancy.

It could be estimated that 10–15% of all women will be concerned by unaesthetic changes to their body after pregnancy, such as abdominal and mammary disfigurement stretchmarks, and general deterioration of the figure. The abdominal wall that will contain and shelter the growing fetus could be seriously damaged by it.

PHYSIOPATHOLOGICAL CAUSES

Pregnancy causes a dramatic distension of the abdominal wall, that involves both the skin and the muscles. The static posture of a pregnant woman is characteristic: the pelvis and the abdomen are pushed forward, while the lumbar region undergoes a hyperlordosis. This stance can become habitual, and is often referred to as 'aesthetic habit' (Fig. 3.5). It is as if the body is leaning backward in an attempt to avoid falling forward, and the abdominal muscles play an essential part in supporting the body weight. These muscles will become very relaxed, starting from the sixth month of pregnancy, due to hormonal influences,

for example, the large rectus muscles may increase up to 6 inches in length. The abdominal wall is distended, the muscles become fatigued, and their weakened areas are dangerously affected. Weight gain causes increased fatigue.

The hormonal phenomenon, the well known hormonal flooding which affects all the tissues of the body, (skin, connective tissue, elastic tissue and fat) is another factor which is implicated in the formation of stretchmarks.

GENERAL APPEARANCE

Pregnancy can leave disfiguring after-effects at different levels of the abdominal wall. The abdominal skin can become distended, wrinkled, creased, and have transverse pleats when the patient is sitting that become worse when she leans forward (Fig. 3.6). This gives the abdomen

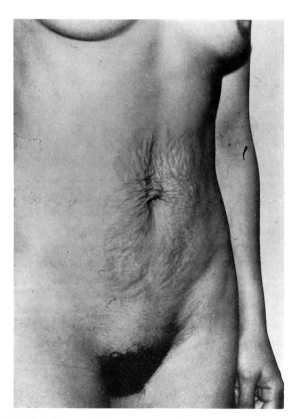

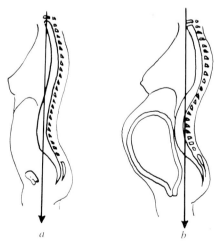

Fig. 3.5 Example of curvature accentation: **a** good static posture; **b** non-corrected in pregnancy under the effect of gravity.

Fig. 3.6 Pre-surgical aspect: wrinkled, stretch marked skin. Central periumbilical lesions (P1); atrophic fat (G2); dehiscant muscular wall (diastasis) (M1).

a 'sagging' appearance, with stretchmarks that differ in number, aspect and topography. These are found mainly on the sides and in the subumbilical region.

Finally, there could be an abdominal scar due to caesarean section. Such scars, after a more or less long hypertrophic phase, remain adherent or umbilicated. In this instance it seems that the quality of the obstetrician's work is much less at fault than the corrective fibroblastic power of the area, which is also under unfavourable hormonal influences.

Fatty tissue

It is well known that the weight gained during pregnancy will not be entirely lost. This phenomenon, in which endocrine and psychological factors play a part, could be responsible for the residual fat on the abdominal wall, giving it a sagging, unpleasant appearance. The muscles can also suffer from being under a long sustained tension, and could emerge very weakened. The resulting lesions involve the weak points of this area. These are:

1. A diastasis of the rectus muscles, corresponding to an enlargement of the linea alba. This diastasis can be functionally uncomfortable and painful. It may be visible, and expressed by the protrusion of the abdominal viscera along an unaesthetic vertical midline from sternum to pubis.
2. An umbilical hernia; this is a weakening of the musculoaponeurotic wall around the umbilical area, and may also be functionally uncomfortable and unaesthetic.

If these are the principal lesions from an analytical point of view, there are three main anatomicoclinical aspects of the abdomen after pregnancy from a synthetic point of view.

Unscathed abdomen

Fortunately, in spite of the above-mentioned problems, the abdomen is undamaged in the majority of cases.

Distended abdomen

This represents the other extreme; here, the damage is very significant and has already been described. It appears as if the whole abdominal wall has collapsed.

Dermal dystrophy

Postgravid dermal dystrophies are found between the two extremes described above. These are withered, creased, stretchmarked and sagging abdomens; the skin looks crumpled. The term 'dermodystrophy' should be used for damage in people of normal figure and weight.

These appearances are variable and depend on the extent, the localization and the association of the different lesions. It is useful to distinguish between localized and dispersed dermal dystrophies.

Localized dermal dystrophies These are either periumbilical, most often with an unpleated umbilicus topped by a pleat or a depression, or they look like supra- or subumbilical pleats; most often they are suprapubic.

Dispersed dermal dystrophies These are associated with a thin, wrinkled skin, covered with pleats that converge towards the umbilicus and leave out the epigastrium. Generally the epigastrium is also affected after a twin pregnancy.

These dermal dystrophies are hardly visible in the standing position, but become much more obvious when the patient sits down or leans forward, and make the wearing of a two-piece swimsuit difficult or impossible! They also make the indication and choice of a surgical technique very difficult. However, they have benefited from many specially designed techniques for localized abdominoplasty with limited cutaneous resection.

Stretchmarks

Stretchmarks are 'fractures' in the elastic fibre of the skin, and are indelible. They are cutaneous weaknesses associated with pregnancy, and have both mechanical and hormonal origins. Distension is a mechanical cause: the stretchmarks of hypertrophic breasts in young people and 'overwork' stretchmarks in sportsmen are evidence of this mechanism.

The hormonal flooding of pregnancy acts at all levels, including the skin, and is enough to cause stretchmarks, as is also the case in some endocrine diseases and in treatments with high doses of steroids. No mechanical factor is necessary in such cases.

Various risk factors involved in the appearance of stretchmarks are:

- Age (below 25)
- Obesity
- Birth of a child over 4 kg
- Being a blond or a redhead
- Rapid weight gain

This last factor and obesity could be controlled by limiting weight gain during pregnancy.

There is no treatment for stretchmarks, since they are true scars of the dermis and thus indelible. Their shape and extent can possibly be alleviated by secondary corrective surgery.

DETERIORATION OF THE FIGURE

Apart from the evident modifications of the belly already described, pregnancy also alters the figure generally, the main reason for this being probably the weight gain that accompanies it. This weight gain is partly physiological and disappears 1–3 months after delivery. However, it is often amplified by bad eating habits. It is important to note that the weight gain due to pregnancy does not correspond to the simple addition of the weight of the fetus + placenta + increase in weight of the uterus + amniotic fluid, which on average adds up to 6 kg. For an ideal weight gain of 11 kg, this leaves 5 kg that corresponds to a real increase in the body weight of the woman, independently of what will be lost during delivery.

This weight gain has both a psychological and an endocrinal origin. Oestrogen increase during pregnancy is the main reason, but psychological parameters play an important part. We know that in some cases, part or all of the weight gained during pregnancy will not be lost afterwards; we know too that obesity frequently starts with pregnancy, or immediately afterwards.

The psychological mechanisms involved are poorly understood. It has been observed that women unconsciously model their eating behaviour on that of the child. Therefore, the abdominal wall and the breasts pay the price of pregnancy via a number of more or less intricate mechanisms:

- Obesity may develop during pregnancy, usually linked to bad eating habits.
- After delivery, the patient may remain fat if she does not rapidly return to a normal body weight.
- Unaesthetic caesarian section scars can mark the abdomen.
- Finally, pregnancy can directly damage the abdominal wall by leaving it creased and stretchmarked. This is characteristic of post pregnancy dermal dystrophies.

However, these lesions, although they are frequent, could be prevented or at least minimized by simple precautions that will be described below.

Prevention

Weight gain should be limited during pregnancy. This is essential both aesthetically and obstetrically. Some simple dietary rules should limit the weight gain to 1 kg per month; thus, a reasonable weight increase would average 9–10 kg, with a maximum of 12–13 kg.

A good abdominal musculature should be maintained. Women should be encouraged to keep up a physical and muscular activity during pregnancy if there is no obstetrical contraindication. Swimming and gymnastics could be very beneficial.

In cases of abnormal vertebral stance that could aggravate an abdominal lesion, physiotherapy could be helpful. However one should be careful with abdominal exercising immediately after delivery, since this could be more harmful than beneficial to the perineal muscles, which will have been very active during delivery. There is a risk of provoking or aggravating perineal lesions that could lead to serious complications such as urinary incontinence.

The wearing of a girdle or a pregnancy belt is not indicated, as it provides a transitory and passive support rather than the physiological muscular support; this will leave the muscles weaker after delivery.

When these preventive measures are ignored, abdominal lesions and pregnancy after-effects do happen; treatment then is essentially surgical.

4. Classification of abdominal wall lesions

It has been seen that female patients undergo abdominal surgery for a variety of reasons, and there are many different operations available. Under the label of abdominoplasty can be included the correction of a pendulous abdomen, correction of periumbilical stretchmarks, excision of excess abdominal fat that does not respond to diet, and excision of abdominal panniculus after the loss of adipose tissue. It would seem worthwhile to classify these abdominal lesions in a clearly logical fashion.

Any classification is, by its very nature, limited and arbitrary, however, classification can be useful in attaining a better grasp of the clinical picture in each individual case prior to surgery, and it can help a great deal in planning the operation.

In order to determine a typical profile of an abdomen, the authors have chosen four parameters corresponding to the four basic elements of abdominal morphology. The clinical study of an abdominal wall prior to surgery should include an appreciation of the skin (S), the subcutaneous fat (F), the condition of the muscles (M), and the general shape of the abdomen (A). Each of these elements will have a coefficient attributed to it, either 0, + or −, depending on its condition. This will enable us to summarize and rapidly synthesize the condition of any abdomen using eight symbols: four to indicate the element concerned and four to evaluate and quantify it. We therefore propose the following methodology to classify the lesions of the abdominal wall.

CONDITION OF THE SKIN (S)

The skin could be normal or subnormal, i.e. with few or no lesions (0).

It could be of very good quality, tonic, elastic and healthy (+).

It could be injured, wrinkled, distended and stretchmarked (−).

CONDITION OF THE SUBCUTANEOUS FAT (F)

The condition of the subcutaneous fat could be normal, intact and smooth (0).

Table 4.1 Classification of abdominal conditions

	0	+	−
Skin (S)	Normal or subnormal, with few or no lesions	Very good quality, elastic and healthy	Injured, wrinkled distended, stretchmarked
Subcutaneous fat (F)	Normal, smooth	Increased, localized or generalized obesity	Atrophic
Muscles (M)	Normal, of normal tonicity	Tonic, strong abdominal wall	Weakened, hernia, eventration, evisceration
General shape of abdomen (A)	Average	Wide	Long

It could be increased in thickness in conditions of generalized or localized obesity (+).

There could be either localized or generalized fat atrophy, especially in the periumbilical area, which in the sitting position gives an unattractive 'bunched up' appearance, with many horizontal folds (−).

CONDITION OF THE MUSCLES (M)

The condition of the muscles could be normal or subnormal, i.e. of normal tonicity (0).

They could be very tonic, with a strong abdominal wall (+).

They could be weakened, in which case diastasis, hernia, eventration or evisceration can be seen (−).

GENERAL SHAPE OF THE ABDOMEN (A)

The abdomen could be wide, with a large ratio of the iliac diameter to the distance between the umbilicus and the pubic triangle (+).

It could be long; in this case the above ratio is small (−).

It could be of intermediary or average shape with a harmonious ratio (0).

Using the symbols described above we can devise a classification that will enable us to schematize the condition of any abdominal wall (Table 4.1). It should be said, however, that this classification has its limitations, but its straightforwardness could be very helpful in planning an operation.

5. Blood and nerve supply to the abdominal wall

THE ARTERIES

The blood supply to the abdominal wall comes from:

1. The superior epigastric, which originates in the sheath of the rectus abdominis and penetrates the muscle mass midway between the xiphoid and the umbilicus.

2. The inferior epigastric artery, originating from the inner side of the external iliac artery, a few millimetres behind and above the inguinal ligament. It goes inwards initially, then curves upwards and inwards. The artery then takes a rising vertical direction, slightly oblique to the umbilicus, thus approaching the rectus sheath. It crosses the outer edge before entering the arch of Douglas. At this point, the artery, now in front of the fascia transversalis, penetrates the sheath of the rectus abdominis muscle.

3. The deep circumflex iliac artery, which comes off the outer aspect of the external iliac artery, at about the level of the epigastric artery. It follows the inguinal ligament, slanting upwards and backwards in the direction of the anterior superior iliac spine. It terminates in the region of the anterior superior iliac spine, and usually has two terminal branches which will anastomose with the abdominal subcutaneous, branches of the lower intercostals, and the lumbar arteries.

4. The superficial epigastric artery, originating from the anterior portion of the femoral artery, just above the crural arch, and ascending through the cribriform fascia to approach the surface. It then continues obliquely upwards and inwards and branches in the subcutaneous tissue up to the area of the umbilicus.

5. The superficial circumflex iliac artery, also originating from the femoral artery, either alone or from a common trunk with the superficial epigastric artery. As with the latter, it penetrates the cribriform fascia to bifurcate in the subcutaneous tissue, but its direction is upwards and outwards. It bypasses the anterosuperior iliac spine to supply the skin of the anterolateral abdominal wall outside the area of the subcutaneous abdominal artery. The terminal branches of these arteries are anastomosed.

6. The lower intercostal arteries, in the upper part. Some branches of the lumbar arteries in the back bring additional blood supply to the abdominal wall.

7. The superficial, external pudendal artery, which supplies a small portion of the lower medial subpubic area.

THE ARTERIAL SYSTEM

The arterial system of the abdominal wall is divided into a deep level and a superficial level. The blood supply of the deep musculo-aponeurotic levels is provided by the epigastric, internal mammary, deep circumflex iliac, intercostal and lumbar arteries. The superficial levels are supplied by the superficial epigastric, superficial circumflex iliac, and the superficial external pudendal arteries, which penetrate the subcutaneous tissue, as well as by other perforating arteries which arise from deeper levels. This quality of blood supply is well shown in the studies undertaken by the authors.

Injecting the entire abdominal wall enabled us to locate the vessels described above and to accurately follow their course and their anastomoses (Fig. 5.1). Briefly, it seems that these vessels run in three directions: a vertical, median direction (the epigastric, internal mammary artery); a superior, external direction (the intercostals); an inferior external direction (the circumflex iliac artery). Moreover, the injections confirmed the richness of the blood supply, especially in the superior and inferior portions of the abdominal wall. In order to find the area of demarcation between the superficial and the deep levels of vessels, it is necessary to carry out an anatomical dissection. When the deep musculoaponeurotic layers are dissected away, there is only skin and fat left, in addition to two large inferior vessels: the abdominal subcutaneous and the superficial circumflex iliac arteries. Apart from these two vessels, the blood supply of the skin and fat of the abdominal wall is provided by the perforating vessels. It is necessary, therefore, to distinguish between the deep or musculoaponeurotic vessels and the superficial or fatty-cutaneous vessels.

Deep blood supply

The deep blood supply comes through the epigastric, internal mammary, deep circumflex iliac, intercostal and lumbar arteries. These have been well described in the past and generally present a constant configuration (Fig. 5.2). A thorough knowledge of this blood supply is essential for abdominal surgery, from the simplest procedure, such as repair of a diastasis recti, to more complicated and demanding operations such as the synthetic repair of an eventration. Two concepts need to be stressed:

1. The anastamosis of the superior epigastric artery to the inferior epigastric artery is variable and sometimes absent, but is

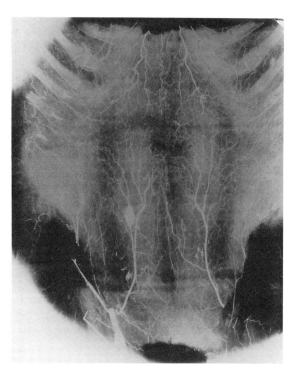

Fig. 5.1 Injection of the entire wall. The vessels go in three directions: a vertical, median direction (the epigastric, internal mammary artery); a superior, external direction (the intercostals); and an inferior-external direction (the circumflex iliac artery).

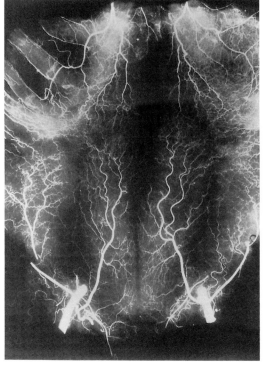

Fig. 5.2 Deep arterial blood supply. The epigastric artery, the deep circumflex iliac artery, the intercostals, and the internal mammary artery can be easily identified.

frequently demonstrated. Generally there is capillary anastomosis in the body of the rectus abdominis.

2. The intercostal arteries play a greater part in the blood supply of the abdominal wall than is generally thought.

From a deductive point of view, it is important to note that because of the circular (centripetal) characteristic of this blood supply, all laparotomy incisions, even combined ones, carry little risk of necrosis of the abdominal wall, unless a portion of the wall is completely detached.

Superficial blood supply

Superficial blood supply is especially important in the viability of abdominal flaps. As we have already seen, there are two superficial arterial suppliers (feeders), the superficial epigastric artery and the superficial circumflex iliac, and the perforating arteries, which come from deeper levels.

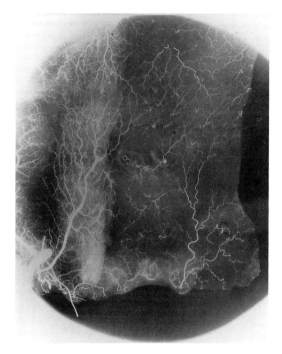

Fig. 5.3 Superficial blood supply. After dissection of the deep musculo-aponeurotic layers, the skin and fat are left in place, and there remain only two large inferior arterial trunks, the superficial iliac circumflex artery and the superficial epigastric artery. Besides these two vessels, the blood supply of the fatty-cutaneous tissue is provided only by the perforating vessels. Note the landmarks of the umbilicus and the left anterosuperior iliac spine.

The inguinocrural area

The large superficial vessels are located in the inguinocrural area. Dissection of the fat layers has shown that these arteries go to the deeper side of the fatty layers. When the adipose tissue is detached at the level of the aponeurosis, the artery can be seen along its entire course without further dissection (Fig. 5.3). These two arteries anastomose with each other, with the last intercostal arteries, and with the ends of the neighbouring perforating arteries, but from a physiological point of view, this is of limited importance. Apart from the two thick arterial trunks, this inguinocrural area has a much sparser blood supply when compared to the abundant network of the perforating arteries.

The perforating arteries

The perforating arteries supply most of the superficial layers, i.e. the fat and skin, of the abdominal wall. They are of vital importance in abdominoplasty, which is concerned with the superficial perforating vessels. It is quite difficult

to reconstruct the lumbar pattern of the perforating arteries by dissection, and for this reason this section is somewhat more vague than the usual anatomical treatises.

For the study of perforating arteries, we used the following technique: the abdominal wall was dissected entirely 24 hours after the injection with radiocorrodan; the muscles and superficial aponeurosis were dissected carefully, while marking the perforating arteries separately (Elbaz, Dardour & Ricbourg 1975). A lead marker was placed at the site of each perforating artery, and a simple roentgenogram of the abdominal wall shows the number and location of these arteries (Fig. 5.4). The results of this study show that there are about 60 perforating arteries from one midaxillary line to the other — 30 on each side — which supply the entire abdominal wall. They are uniformly located in the abdominal wall. A

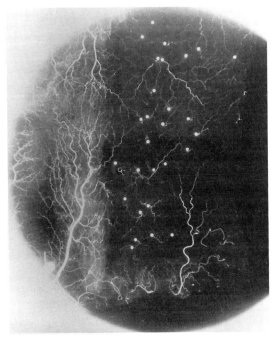

Fig. 5.4 The perforating arteries. Roentgenogram of one half of the abdominal wall, after marking each perforating artery with a lead marker.

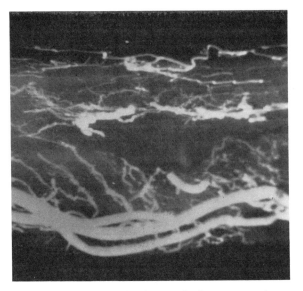

Fig. 5.5 Studies of perforating arteries in a cross-section of the total abdominal wall through roentgenography show these arteries forming a candelabra-shaped termination. They cross all levels, creating sinous trunks with fat globules in the form of a net, and spread out in the form of a subdermal plexus at the deeper side of the of the chorionic layer, and then in another supradermal, subpapillar plexus, which is more superficial and not as richly supplied.

closer look will reveal an area near the lower arterial trunks which is devoid of perforating arteries. The length of the perforating arteries varies from 2 to 6 cm, the width is about 1 mm.

Another study shows that all the perforating arteries anastomose on a level parallel with the skin, and that they constitute a subdermal plexus of vessels which radiate around the umbilicus. There are two observations to be made on this arterial network:

1. If the perforating arteries are fairly evenly distributed, the density of their loops varies according to the area. The density is greatest in the periumbilical and subcostal areas, and very sparse in the subumbilical area.

2. Often, the superficial epigastric artery and the superficial circumflex iliac artery anastomose in the main corridor of the perforating arteries, although this is not common. Most interesting is the way in which the perforating arteries terminate, which is seen in the cross-sections of the total

abdominal wall on X-ray study (Fig. 5.5). Therefore, we see that the perforating arteries, which run vertically, form networks through all levels with the adipose cells and spread out to form a subdermal plexus on the underside of the chorion, and then a rich supradermal or a less rich subpapillary plexus, which is more superficial. This arrangement of perforating arteries is homogeneous on the entire abdominal wall (Fig. 5.6).

These arciform anastomoses, which are parallel to the skin surfaces, join with neighbouring perforators to enrich the dermal plexuses.

The cutaneous blood supply can be outlined in the following manner:

1. The network perpendicular to the skin surface, perforating the dermal layers from the deepest to the most superficial.

2. The superficial network parallel to the skin, the dermal plexuses and the supra- and subdermal plexuses.

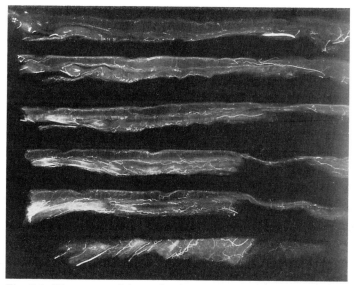

Fig. 5.6 The pattern of the perforating arteries as well as that of the supra- and subdermal plexuses is uniform throughout the abdominal wall.

SURGICAL CONCLUSIONS

Certain surgical conclusions can be drawn from this knowledge of anatomy.

If the defatting of a portion of a flap is theoretically dangerous, the presence of a subpapillary network of vessels explains, under certain conditions, how a portion of defatted skin can survive. An example of this is the 'defatted Colson flap'.

The level of detachment must be deep in order to maintain the subdermal network, but practically speaking, it is preferable to leave a thin layer of fat on the aponeurosis to avoid retraction of the perforating arteries behind the aponeurosis while they are being cut. This will also make haemostasis easier (Figs 5.7, 5.8).

ARTERIAL HAEMODYNAMICS OF THE FATTY CUTANEOUS PANNICULUS

Two cases will be compared, one in which the superficial panniculus is detached from the deep musculoaponeurotic layer, and one in which it is not.

When the abdominal wall is in place, the arterial blood supply is assured by the perforating arteries, which bring blood from the deeper net-

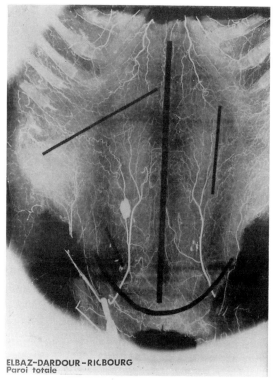

ELBAZ-DARDOUR-RICBOURG
Paroi totale

Fig. 5.7 Projection of the most frequent approaches to the abdomen. One can easily conceive that the midline incision may not be given to haemorrhage and that, on the contrary, a right subcostal, lateral or Pfannenstiel incision needs much more careful haemostasis.

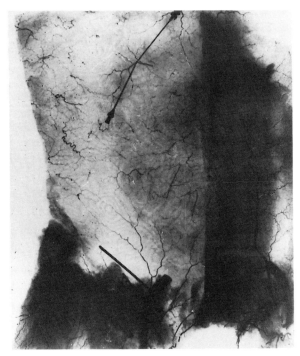

Fig. 5.8 A roentgenogram of an abdominal wall which was injected, and which shows two old scars: one subcostal and one appendectomy scar marked here with radio-opaque material. These two scars are invisible on the roentgenogram, even with magnification. They have been revascularized by the subdermal capillary network.

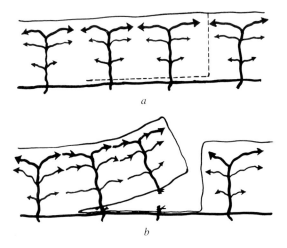

Fig. 5.9 Outline of the arterial haemodynamics of the fatty-cutaneous tissue of the abdominal wall. **a** The abdominal wall in place. Multicentric vascularization is due to the perforating arteries in the shape of a chandelier. The dotted line marks the area to be detached. **b** A section of the fatty-cutaneous wall is detached; note the ligating perforating arteries. The blood supply becomes 'one way.' The subdermal arched network, as well as the sub- and supradermic capillary plexus become very important.

works. Each perforating artery has its own area to supply, that is, a multicentric vascularization. The richness of the blood supply at this deep level, and its centrifugal pattern with regard to the umbilicus, lead one to believe that lesions appearing at this level have no impact on the blood supply of the skin.

When a fatty-cutaneous segment is detached, the blood supply for this area comes only from the peripheral perforating arteries. The multicentric circulation then becomes a one-way street, that is, a 'terminal', and the importance of a subdermal network in the arches and the subdermal and supradermal capillary plexus can be seen (Fig. 5.9).

VEINS OF THE ABDOMINAL WALL

The importance of the veins of the abdominal wall is significant, since venous return is absol-

utely necessary to the survival of an abdominal flap. Yet the study of the venous system shows that it is complex, not so much in its extremely variable anatomy, but in its physiology. Attempts to inject the superficial venous network have failed, even when attempted directly and under pressure, with the abdominal subcutaneous and the superficial circumflex iliac veins. The veins, like the arteries, are in two levels, the superficial fatty-cutaneous level and the deep musculoaponeurotic level.

Deep level

As in the arterial system, the deep venous level remains remarkably constant. Moreover, it is easy to inject it against its flow, which simplifies its study. The venous system approximates that of the arterial; there are two veins for each artery. The inferior drainage is carried out by the epigastric and the deep circumflex iliac veins, which drain into the external iliac veins. The epigastric veins can receive a collateral drainage directly from the umbilicus.

All these veins are united by many anastomoses, both small and large, which appear clearly during the dissection of the major muscle mass. The superior and inferior intercaval anastomoses are completed by a portocaval anastomosis at the level of the umbilicus.

Superficial or fatty-cutaneous level

This network is not strictly superimposable on the arterial one. It is impossible to inject this network against its flow, and that explains why it is poorly described in the literature. The best description was given by Poirier, who took it from Braune: it is a network with elongated loops which unite the axillary veins and those of the neck and the thighs, and which contains many valves. Poirier describes the veins as follows:

1. The abdominal subcutaneous or tegumentous veins of the abdomen.
2. The subcutaneous iliac veins, often double, flowing into the femoral veins.
3. The subcutaneous thoracoepigastric vein, which unites the femoral to the axillary vein on the outer side of the abdomen.
4. The median subcutaneous xiphoid vein originating near the umbilicus, where it anastomoses with the paraumbilical vein.

RESULTS OF STUDY

Based on these classic points, our dissection differed in certain respects. There are many anatomical variations; the veins can be very large compared to the arteries. On the other hand, they can be very frail and almost non-existent, except microscopically. The venous return in these cases is assured by the subdermal plexus. The superficial epigastric vein or tegumentous vein can be simple, or it can form two or three branches of origin which converge toward a thick trunk (3–4 mm in diameter), emptying into the arch of the saphenous vein. This vein is constant, but even so, its route is rarely comparable to that of the artery. The superficial circumflex iliac vein can be simple or duplicated, voluminous or frail, or can be absent. The thoracoepigastric vein did not appear to be constant.

Through the dissection of the fatty tissue, we were able to locate precisely the parietal veins. The arteries originated at the deepest level of the fatty-cutaneous tissue, but the veins were superficial, located immediately beneath the skin. These two levels are often indiscernible in a lean abdominal wall. On the whole, the superficial fatty-cutaneous vascularization is extremely variable, and many flaps which appear to be dependent on vascularity depend in fact on a subdermal plexus.

Drainage

There are four methods of drainage:

1. From the superficial to the deep layers when the fatty-cutaneous tissue has not been detached from the deep level.
2. Towards the internal mammary plexus and the intercostal one, in the supraumbilical abdomen.
3. Towards the internal saphenous for the subumbilical region.
4. Towards the umbilicus in order to reach the epigastric veins and the paraumbilical vein when this is permeable.

When this last pathway is forced against the flow, the result is stasis with a collateral circulation, an example of which would be the 'jelly fish head' of Cruveillier–Baumgarten cirrhosis.

This one-way venous return explains why, in an anterior lipectomy, the subumbilical point lowered to the pubis is the one that suffers most, since poor venous return is aggravated by the stretching that compresses and crushes the veins.

After all these anatomical considerations, it is clear that the arterial and venous plexuses are of great importance. In most cases, the plexus is capable of becoming permeable again; a subcostal scar is not, therefore, a contraindication to abdominal lipectomy, as long as the scar is 1 year old or more.

NERVES OF THE ANTEROLATERAL ABDOMINAL WALL (Fig. 5.10)

The anterolateral abdominal wall is innervated by the six lower intercostal nerves and other ab-

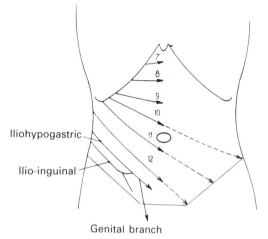

Fig. 5.10 Nerves of the anterior lateral abdominal wall. It is innervated by the lower 6 intercostal nerves and the abdomino-genitals. They all stop on the anterior midline. The dotted lines continue their dissection until their reference mark. (According to C. Gouinaud, Anatomie de l'abdomen, Doin, Paris).

abdominis sheath. Their direction is variable: the seventh proceeds upwards and inwards, the eighth and the ninth are practically horizontal, and the last four proceed downwards. They follow a pathway from a point 1 cm below the anterior end of the corresponding rib, to the anterior superior iliac spine on the opposite side for the tenth intercostal nerve; to the middle of the inguinal ligament on the opposite side for the 11th; to the pubic spine on the opposite side for the 12th.

Before reaching the external margin of the rectus abdominis sheath, each nerve divides into 15 minor branches, forming important plexuses between the large muscles. These proceed towards the deep side of the rectus abdominis then reach the external half of the muscle.

Different nerves innervate different muscular segments: the seventh intercostal nerve runs to the superior segment, the eighth nerve runs to the second segment, and the 11 and 12th nerves run to the fourth segment. Terminal branches provide the sensitive innervation of the abdominal wall and give rise to a lateral branch that supplies its anterolateral portion.

dominal nerves. These intercostal nerves are located in the abdominal wall between the transversis abdominis and the internal oblique, thus reaching the external margin of the rectus

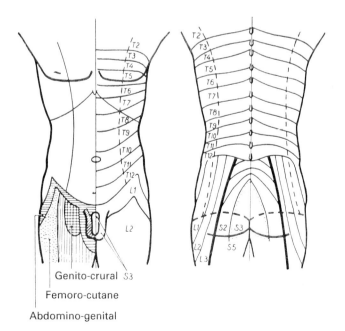

Fig. 5.11 Sensitive innervation of the abdominal wall. (According to Dejerine in C. Gouinard, Anatomie de l'abdomen, Doin, Paris).

Finally, anatomists have described a nerve that supplies different abdominal muscles through its abdominal branch; they called this the 'abdominogenital nerve'.

MOTOR INNERVATION OF THE ANTEROLATERAL ABDOMINAL WALL MUSCLES

Rectus abdominis

This is innervated by the terminal branches of the six lower intercostal nerves, the iliohypogastric nerve and the ilio-inguinal nerve.

The triangular pyramidalis muscle

This is innervated by the 12th intercostal and the iliohypogastric nerve.

External oblique

This is supplied by the perforating branches of the six lower intercostal nerves, the iliohypogastric and ilio-inguinal nerves.

Internal oblique and transversus abdominis

These are innervated by the lower four intercostal nerves and the iliohypogastric and ilio-inguinal nerves.

All these nerves form a rich plexus that largely supplies the abdominal wall. A paralysis will not occur unless at least two consecutive nerves are sectioned.

SENSITIVE INNERVATION AND DERMATOMES OF THE ANTEROLATERAL ABDOMINAL WALL (Fig. 5.11)

There are numerous plexus formations and important distributions of peripheral fibres. Therefore, surgical incisions that resect nerve trunks can only provoke transitory anaesthesia (approximately 6 months).

6. The lymphatic system of the abdominal wall

'In the present age of high technology one of the primary challenges to studying lymphatics is to find them'. Kanter M. A. 1987 Plastic and Reconstructive Surgery 79; 131–139

A good anatomical and physiological knowledge of the lymphatic system is essential for a better understanding of the surgical techniques of abdominoplasty.

The detachment or undermining of the superior abdominal flap entails a distortion of the superficial lymphatic system. The lymphatic system can be responsible for the development of complications following abdominoplasty: for example, the possible growth of a seroma, which is probably a parietal liquid discharge of lymphatic origin and an oedema of the superior flap. After reviewing the anatomical points, brief mention will be made of the conclusions of a personal study by the authors, consisting of a series of in vivo lymphatic dissections. Finally the lymphatic healing process will be considered, in order to study the formation of seromas.

ANATOMY

The superficial lymphatics originating in the skin should be distinguished from the deep lymphatics originating in the musculoaponeurotic plane. The lymphatic channels and terminal lymph nodes for each territory will be described.

Superficial lymphatics

Lymphatic course

There are distinct supraumbilical and subumbilical territories. The supraumbilical territory has an ascending drainage towards the axillar lymph nodes. The epigastric region is very rich in lymphatics; this is a well known fact and clinically a substantial lymphatic discharge can often be seen after a major abdominoplasty. The supraumbilical lymphatic vessels form two large trunks that converge toward the axillary region and end in the external mammary lymph nodes.

The subumbilical territory drains into the superficial inguinal nodes. The subumbilical lymphatic system is not as dense as the supraumbilical one. The umbilicus drains into the superficial inguinal nodes.

According to Rouvière (1981, 1984), the division between the supraumbilical and the subumbilical territories is a horizontal line running from the umbilicus to L2–L3, but according to Poirier, Cunéo and Marcille, this line is even higher and thus considerably reduces the axillary participation in the lymphatic drainage of the superior flap in an abdominoplasty. This higher limit explains why a low transverse abdominal incision that interrupts the lymphatic drainage towards the inguinal folds, could provoke postoperative lymphatic complications.

No lymphatic anastomosis has ever been described between the supraumbilical and the subumbilical territories, or between the territories on either side of the midline.

Terminal nodes

The terminal lymph nodes of the superficial lymph system of the abdominal wall belong to the superficial axillary and inguinal groups. The external mammary chain drains the supraumbilical skin, and the superficial inguinal lymph nodes

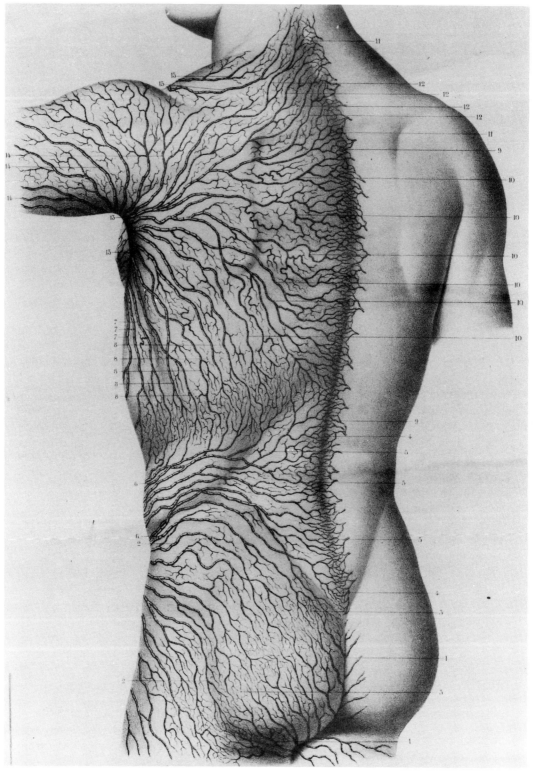

a

Fig. 6.1 Lymphatic system of the trunk. (According to Sappey). **a** Vessels of the posterior wall; **b** vessels of the anterior and lateral walls. They converge towards the axillar and inguinal lymph nodes.

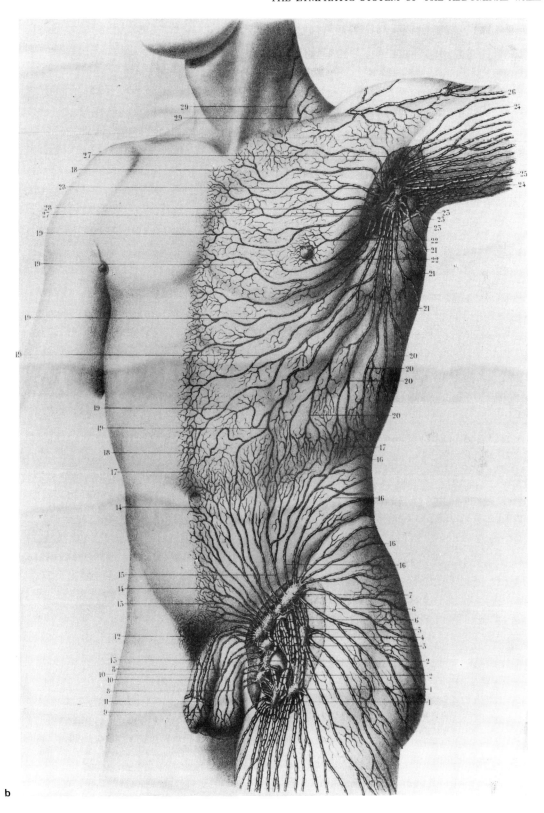

b

drain the subumbilical skin. Located in Scarpa's triangle, these lymph nodes occupy the subcutaneous tissue between the superficial fascia and the aponeurosis. The superior groups can be divided into an external group and an internal group.

The superior external lymph nodes follow the superficial circumflex iliac vessels. The superior internal nodes follow the superficial epigastric vessels and the external pudendal artery. Efferent tubules emerge from the inguinal lymph nodes that go directly to either the external iliac nodes or to the retroinguinal nodes.

Deep lymphatics

These drain the parietal muscles and their aponeurosis. They are not injured in an abdominoplasty unless it is associated with the treatment of ventral hernia.

Lymphatic course

The deep lymphatics follow the blood vessels; three main trunks can be distinguished: the epigastric trunk; the deep circumflex iliac trunk — these both reach the retroinguinal iliac nodes; the satellite trunks of the abdominal branch of the internal mammary vessels. These reach the internal mammary nodes.

The deep lymphatic drainage system of the abdominal muscles can easily be imagined. The rectus abdominis and its sheath depend on the internal mammary chains in the supraumbilical area and on the inferior epigastric one in the subumbilical area. The oblique muscles and the transversus abdominis depend on the epigastric chain, and the umbilical region depends on a complex drainage system consisting of the epigastric chains, the lumbar trunks in the back, and the intraperitoneal nodes near the round ligament and the urachus.

Terminal nodes

These are the retrosternal internal mammary nodes and the retrocrural nodes belonging to the external iliac chains.

There is no communication between the superficial and the deep lymphatics. Just one communication was found located 2 cm above the umbilicus in the midline (Fig. 6.1a,b).

EXPERIMENTAL WORK

The authors have studied the lymphatic system of various abdominoplasty patients. The lymphatic circulation can be visualized using the Hudack method, with in vivo intradermic injections of patent violet blue. This dye has the unique property of being selectively absorbed by the lymphatics. After a careful dissection it was possible to identify the lymphatics and to follow their course; no lymphography was carried out because of the high risk of embolism (Figs. 6.2, 6.3).

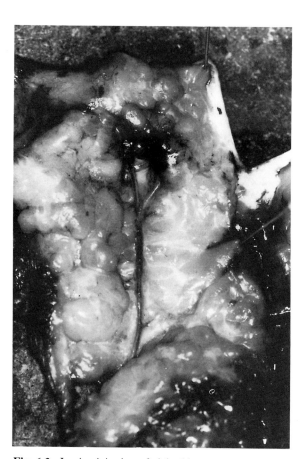

Fig. 6.2 In vivo injection of violet blue-patent. Visualization of a lymphatic vessel in the deep fatty tissue.

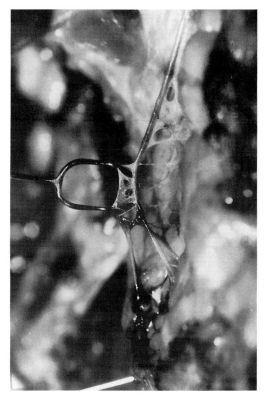

Fig. 6.3 Injection of a lymphatic trunk.

Results

The authors' conclusions are a little different from the classic descriptions:

1. The limit between the superior and inferior lymphatic territories seems to be much lower than previously thought. It follows a horizontal line located halfway between the umbilicus and the pubis.
2. It was possible to determine the relationship between the superficial lymphatics and the superficial fascia. The main lymphatic vessels are found in the fatty layer (reticular or lamellar layer) immediately beneath the superficial fascia.
3. The superficial lymphatic trunks were seen to follow the vascular courses. Their size is variable, up to 4 mm in diameter. They have a straight course, except in the obese patient.
4. The lymphatic circulation is fast, and is slowed down only by some very few nodes

situated in the superficial fatty layer. It took an extremely short time for the dye to appear 10 cm away from the point of injection.
5. No perforating lymphatics were identifiable on either side of the fascia or the aponeurosis; this could be due to an experimental error.
6. It was possible, however, to see some important lymphatic communications between the areas on either side of the midline (classically these were considered minimal).
7. The richness of the lymphatic system is not proportional to that of the vascular system.

Critical analysis

These observations should be viewed with caution, since:

1. There are different anatomical variations in the lymphatic system from one individual to another.
2. With the method of injection used, only the superficial lymphatic system and not the deep one can be visualized.
3. The functional circulation does not follow the classic anatomical description of the lymphatic courses. This is why the injection of cadavers (Gerota method) does not give the same dynamic results as the method described above.
4. Finally, there could have been artefacts due to the experimental method used: any obstacle (compression, ligature) on the lymphatic course could reverse the normal flow.

THE LYMPHATIC HEALING PROCESS

It has never been possible to histologically observe the healing process of a sectioned lymphatic canal, but lymphography has formally proved the reestablishment of a functional flow. The hypothesis of a neogenesis or regeneration has been mentioned in passing.

Physiological review

Lymphostasis

Lymphostasis is the first healing step following the resection of a lymphatic canal. The lymph is able to coagulate spontaneously; its coagulation is slower than that of blood, because of its lower concentration in fibrinogen and prothrombin, and the chemical composition of the lymph is different from one site to another. In vitro, the lymph coagulates in 20–40 minutes.

With fibrin glue (fibrinogen and thrombin) a fibrin clot can be obtained in 30 seconds to 3 minutes.

Cellular healing

Lymphatic healing requires a correct immobilization of the edges. The repositioning of the superior flap over the superficial side of the aponeurosis is essential. It had been thought that by keeping a thin fatty layer over the aponeurosis, lymphostasis became easier; opinions have since changed on this: the healing process is actually easier with fatty-fatty layers than with fatty-aponeurotic ones.

Restitutio ad integrum

Lymphatic healing does not lead to a restitutio ad integrum: restoration of the smooth fibres of the lymphatics does not occur. Regeneration of the lymphatic valves remains a hypothesis.

Medicosurgical means

Surgical ligature and electrocoagulation could achieve lymphostasis of the big trunks. Compressive postoperative dressings or elasticated sheaths will immobilize the different edges. Biological glues are also very helpful, having both a biological and a mechanical action in that they reinforce the lymphatic coagulation and facilitate the repositioning of the superior flap by eliminating the dead space. Lymphatic drainage can also be used to treat any oedema of the superior flap due to lymphatic stasis.

7. Mechanical properties and ageing of the abdominal wall

Apart from cases of major trauma to the musculoaponeurotic fascia, changes in the abdominal wall, whether they are connected with obesity, pregnancy, or ageing, can involve the skin and subcutaneous tissue, which are rich in fat cells. Molecular biology and the progress of biochemistry have completely changed the classic concepts of medicine regarding connective tissue. Recent and conclusive studies enable us to better understand the pathological and degenerative processes of connective tissue, which account for more than 70% of the mortality and morbidity in the western world today.

The advent of liposuction, with its mandatory preoperative assessment of the mechanical qualities of the skin, gives even more importance to this chapter. There follows a brief review of the main characteristics of the connective tissue and its normal and pathological metabolism.

CONNECTIVE TISSUE

Whatever the histological differences in connective tissue may be, whether in the blood vessels, the cartilage or the adipose tissue of the abdominal wall, the common elements are cellular (fibrocytes, fibroblasts, adipose cells, histiocytes, macrophages) and an intracellular matrix made up of four types of macromolecules which give the connective tissue its mechanical properties. These macromolecules include collagen, elastin, proteoglycans (complex protein–mucopolysaccharide acids corresponding to the reticulofibrous cells which we classically study), and the structural glycoproteins (fundamental substances which are the basis for cells and fibres).

The regulation of the relative speeds of production of these four substances conditions their respective densities, a major factor in the differentiation of the various connective tissues; for example, all tendons are rich in collagen, the aorta is rich in elastin, and cartilage is rich in glycoprotein.

Collagen and elastin have a fundamental mechanical role and are directly involved in the pathology of the abdominal wall. Hence, ageing of the skin is characterized by lesions specifically involving the collagen fibres and the elastic tissues; it is for this reason that stress will be laid upon these two elements of connective tissue, in the light of recent studies.

COLLAGEN

Collagen is one of the most widely studied molecules today. It can be found in almost all types of connective tissue, and itself accounts for about one-third of the body's protein. Collagen fibres, which never anastomose, are found in the direction of the strongest pull which will be exerted on the tissues.

Structure of collagen

Each collagen fibre is formed of a bundle of parallel fibres. Under the ordinary microscope, using polarized light, these fibrils show a positive birefringence, i.e. an orientation. Examined under the electronic microscope, they seem to consist of a juxtaposition of filaments which present with a periodic cross-striation of 640 Å; this periodicity is characteristic of collagen. These filaments are themselves made up of a juxtaposition of proto-fibrils, formed by three polypeptide chains rolled into the shape of a helix (triple helicoid).

Chemical constitution

Among the aminoacids making up the collagen molecule, one-third is glycocoll, one-third proline, and one-third hydroxyproline. Such an abundance of hydroxyproline is typical of collagen.

Biosynthesis

Aminoacids renew themselves slowly; thus, when studying the prospects of injected radioactive glycocoll and the speed of fixation in newly formed collagen, it has been possible to measure a daily rate of renewal of 0.5–3%. It is now known that there are five genetically different collagens; their sequential synthesis in certain tissues can be ascribed to the repression and activation of their structure-coding genes.

One of the most important traits in the biosynthesis of this protein seems to be the existence of post-transcriptional reactions which intervene in its synthesis and secretion. These reactions are the hydroxylation of lysine and proline, followed by collagen bridging, which is essential in the formation of a tridimensional fibrous network having sufficient mechanical resistance. Recent studies have shown that inflammatory collagen, produced in scars and granulation tissue, has a type of bridging different from that of normal collagen and similar to that of embryonic collagen. In the normal scarring process, the bridging of the collagen tissue is of an adult type, whereas in hypertrophic scars, for example, the bridging is of an embryonic type.

ELASTIN

Elastin has long been a mystery, and is apparently inert. It is now beginning to attract a great deal of attention. It has been proven that the progressive degeneration of elastic fibre plays a great part in the ageing of connective tissues, both at the arterial level and at the level of the skin. Elastin is the body's elastic protein. Its fibres can stretch up to 120% of their initial length, and then return to their original length in the resting state. The fibres anastomose in a network of very wide loops, in smooth or arched blades.

Structure of elastin

Under an ordinary microscope with polarized light, the elastic fibres are birefringent when stretched. Under an electronic microscope they do not demonstrate any periodic cross-striation. Proelastin, the precursor of elastin, has recently been isolated; it undergoes a series of reactions leading to bridging, and then becomes rubber-like (Robert 1974, 1975).

Chemical–physical composition

Elastin is a resistant protein that is insoluble in water, saline, acid or base solutions. It is specifically attacked by elastase, a pancreatic extract recently demonstrated in blood platelets, in polynuclear, and in the arterial wall itself. It contains the same quantity of glycocoll as collagen (one-third), but it lacks the hydroxyproline which is characteristic of collagen.

Biosynthesis

We have seen how proelastin undergoes a series of reactions leading to its bridging, which makes it the elastic protein of the body. This vulcanization depends on one enzyme, lysine-oxidase, which has been isolated and purified. Robert and his colleagues at the Biochemical Laboratory of Connective Tissue at Creteil, have proved, by using tissue cultures of the aorta, that there is a regulation of the relative speeds of biosynthesis of the macromolecular components of the arterial wall, depending on the age of the subject. Moreover, these studies have stressed the existence of an active biosynthesis of elastin in adults, contrary to what had long been thought.

Reactions of elastin and elastase with calcium and lipids

It has long been known that arterial ageing is characterized by a progressive calcification of the arterial wall, with infiltration of lipids and a subsequent loss of elasticity. Thrombosis has often complicated these changes. This process seems irreversible and affects most human beings. It is not limited to the vascular walls: Bouissou and colleagues (1973) demonstrated that the progressive destruction of elastic fibres was especially important in the coronary arteries. Here, the slightly delayed second phase affected the walls of the large vessels and the elastic tissue of the skin. Recent progress in the biochemistry of connective tissue enables us to better understand the ageing of connective tissue, its pathology, and the degeneration of elastic fibre.

Elastase, which is released from the platelets, the leucocytes and the cells of the abdominal wall, begins the fragmentation of the elastic fibre. A peptide of elastin, due to its tridimensional structure, fixes the calcium very strongly. The lipoproteins, crossing the vessel walls, bring in lipids which adhere to elastic fibres, because of

their affinity for these hydrophobic and lipophilic chains. These phenomena seem to be stressed and accelerated by an autoimmune mechanism of atherogenesis. It is therefore easy to understand that these elastic fibres, heavy with lipidocalcium complexes, lose their essential property and degenerate rapidly, first by fragmentation and later by complete lysis (Fig. 7.1).

AGEING OF THE SKIN

Study methodology

Bouissou, in his work on the deltoid skin, the aorta and the coronary arteries, was especially interested in the ageing of the skin and its relationship with concomitant changes in the vessel walls. The method of his study was as follows: skin samples measuring 1×1.5 cm were excised from the deltoid area during autopsy of 241 subjects, ranging in age from 20 to 85 years.

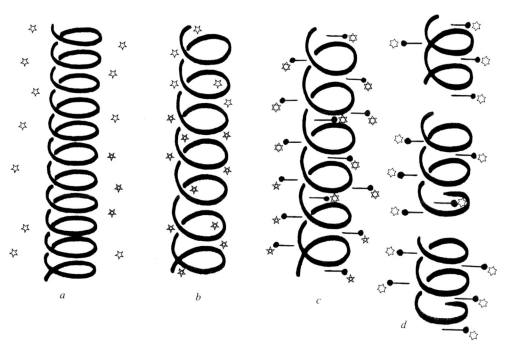

Fig. 7.1 Diagram of the formation lipid deposits on the elastic fibres (from Jacotot and Robert). **a** The elastic fibre is represented as a lipophile and hydrophobe, excluding the molecules of water from its vicinity. **b** The stretching of the fibres changes their relationship to the water of the environment, which causes them to return to their original length (rubber-like elasticity). **c** Lipids are brought into the vessel walls by lipoproteins in transit and enter into the turns of the elastic loops because of their affinity for these hydrophobic peptides. **d** The result is a loss of elasticity and an accelerated degradation.

Excisions were made with a LaGrot blade, and preparation was made for a study of the collagen and elastic fibres. Two samples were taken from the level of the aorta and the right coronary artery for study. The authors proposed to study normal skin, aged skin, and the relationships between ageing of the skin and of the arteries and arteriosclerosis.

Together with Mitz and Vilde, the authors of this book decided to study the state of the dermo-elastic network with reference to cutaneous lipodystrophies and the problems of the figure in general. The study involved 21 subjects, and comprised 12 mammoplasties, seven abdomino-plasties and two trochanteric lipectomies. The average age of the subjects was 31.8 years. Excisions of the epidermis, dermis and hypodermis were performed; samples of skin marked by the surgeon were avoided.

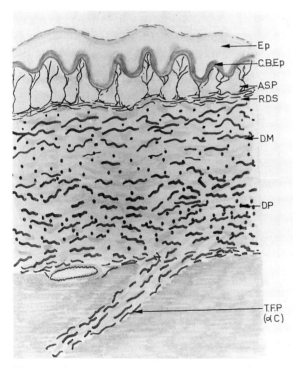

Fig. 7.2 Outline of the elastic tissue of normal skin. The elastic fibres are dark. Ep, epidermis; CBEp, basic layer of the epidermis; ASP subpapillary arborizations, RDS, superficial dermal network; DM, median skin; DP, deep skin; TFP, deep fibrous spans.

The samples were prepared histologically with a thickness of 5 μ, after paraffin solution. The results will be described in three sections, the normal aspect of dermal elastic tissue; the biomechanics of normal and pathological skin; and classification of the lesions.

Normal skin

The normal aspect of dermal elastic tissue can be outlined in five topographical sections from the surface to the deepest level (Fig. 7.2).

1. Subpapillar arborization (SPA). This is a network of long and very frail elastic fibres that ends at the deep side of the papillary epidermis and the cutaneous connections. These fibres diverge in elegant tree shapes from the superficial dermal networks and rise perpendicularly to the skin.
2. The superficial dermal network (SDN). This constitutes the second layer, and is formed by many very thin networks, which interchange fibres. The latter are long, fine, and lie parallel to the skin. The most superficial fibres of the second layer send out papillary branches, shaped as narrow fibres jutting out perpendicularly from the level of the skin and ending at the deep side of the epidermal membrane, as has already been seen. Layers 1 and 2 form the superficial skin.
3. The third layer is the papillary skin of Bouissou, or median skin (MS). It is a thick and dense layer. At this level there is a very important collagen matrix in which the elastic fibres form many netlike networks, thus giving the collagen its specific structure. The cuts show that there are several more levels of elastic network, made of thicker fibres, than in the first two layers. The total network contains several layers. This dermal tissue takes on a sandwich-like structure, which can extend in all directions, yet retains a strong tendency to return to its original shape, although we must take into account at this point the thickness of the median skin.
4. The fourth layer is the subpapillary layer of Bouissou, or deep skin (DS). It is as thick and dense as the median skin and its geostructure

is similar. There are alternating reticular layers of elastic fibres from the depths to the surface, whose main directions change from one layer to the other, feeding a collagen matrix penetrated by many capillary loops. The deep side of the dermal layer is different at the level of the breast and the abdomen; it sends down cordlike fibres which run vertical or oblique to the skin. These fibres constitute the framework of the deep fibrous spans of the hypodermis.

5. The fifth layer is made up of the deep fibrous spans (DFS). We have seen how these fibres originate from the deep skin and then cross the hypodermis, which is thus divided into fat-cell compartments. The deep layers of the skin are therefore solidly anchored to the superficial fascia, and on the aponeurotic level by these true dermal ligaments. The histological structure is peculiar: it includes a matrix of collagen fibres crossed by elastic bundles parallel to the direction of the span. At the centre of this span an arteriovenous axis and a sensory nerve are found, which make up a superficial perforating pedicle for the skin.

It should be noted that the fibres of the superficial and deep layers (layers 1 and 5 respectively) perpendicular to the level of the skin, frame the fibres of the three intermediary layers, whose general direction is parallel to the skin. The third and fourth layers, consisting of a collagen matrix and strengthened by elastic fibres, are the thickest and the most resistant from a mechanical point of view.

BIOMECHANICS OF NORMAL AND PATHOLOGICAL SKIN

Analysing the morphology of the different elastic layers of the skin leads to the following biomechanical interpretation.

The first layer of the skin, made of subpapillary arborizations perpendicular to the skin, attaches the epidermis to the dermis. Thus it contributes to the ability of the epidermis to slide on its supports, and ensures an elastic return while avoiding excessive detachment.

The second layer gives rise to the elastic fibres which form the SPA and constitute the root of the first layer. Moreover, it is joined on its deepest side to the third layer, or median skin. The first and second layers therefore represent a specialized portion of the skin, which ensures the stability of the epidermis on the dermis.

The third layer, or median skin, is specific to the dermis. It is the most solid framework of the skin and represents its essential properties. This level sees the most obvious damage from mechanical lesions; for example, stretchmarks are generally connected with the pseudoarthroses which mostly affect this area.

The fourth layer, or deep skin, is made up of elastic fibres and a collagen matrix whose pattern and direction are comparable to those found in the third layer. Thus, when it is damaged, there are generally lesions just above it. Such damage, however, indicates the seriousness of the lesion. The diversity of orientation of these fibres, which comprise each level of this layer, seems to be protected in the case of unidirectional stretching. This layer gives rise to the deep fibrous span on its deep side.

The fifth layer is formed by the deep fibrous spans of the abdomen, which affix the dermis to the deep aponeurotic layer. The fatty panniculus is divided by these fibrous attachments into fatty cushions, on which the dermis rolls. A major mechanical distension can cause lesions of these fibrous spans, detaching the skin from its deepest moorings.

The biomechanics of normal skin are unique. The skin is a heterogeneous tissue in which each of the five layers plays a specific part of anchoring the epidermis; anchoring in depth the elastic network and providing multidirectional protection.

CLASSIFICATION OF LESIONS

Bouissou and his colleagues, in their work on the deltoid skin, studied changes in the dermal elastic network due to ageing. The lesions described allowed the authors to outline the different stages of ageing of the elastic tissue and to set up a very clear and useful classification. There are four stages of increasing gravity (0, I, II and III); however, the importance of the destruction of elastic fibres in the authors' studied samples led to the addition of a stage IV.

Stage 0: normal
Stage I
Subpapillary arborizations: little or no damage
Superficial skin network: little or no change
Median and deep skin: some cracks at the level of the normal layers
Deep fibrous spans: a few cracks, but the number of elastic fibres is homogeneous
Stage II
SPA: invisible
SDN: frail but visible and with few fractures
MS: very damaged (fractures +++)
DS: little damage (some fractures)
DFS: many fractures but the direction is visible and the fibres have a good density
Stage III
SPA: invisible
SDN: some elastic fibres are still visible
MS and DS: many fractures but the density of the elastic fibres is still very good
DFS: very many fractures but the number of fibres is still high

Stage IV
SPA: invisible
SDN: invisible
MS and DS: micropunctated but not dense
DFS: elastic fibres are rare and very short (fractures +++)

These are the different ageing stages of the elastic tissue (Fig. 7.3).

Two important points from the studies of Bouissou and his group must be stressed:

1. The 45th year seems to be critical for ageing, since dermal lesions and stage II and III changes seem to be frequent after that age.
2. There is an unquestionable chronological parallel between the ageing of the elastic tissue in skin and that of the arterial walls. These dermal elastic tissue lesions are identical with those appearing in the same subjects in the wall of the aorta. Coronary lesions appear somewhat earlier (Fig. 7.4).

It seems, then, that the network of elastic fibres plays an essential part both in the mechanical properties of connective tissue and in the process of ageing and degeneration which it undergoes.

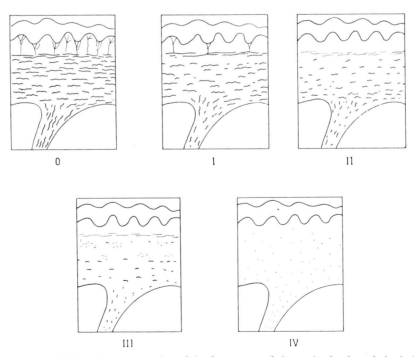

Fig. 7.3 Schematic representation of the four stages of change in the dermal-elastic fibres.

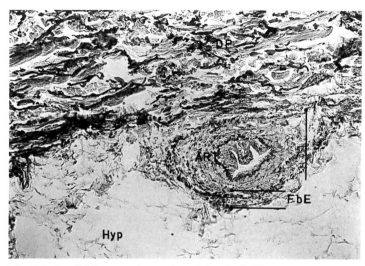

Fig. 7.4 Parallel between destruction of the elastic fibers of the dermis and the damage to the elastic network of a subdermal arteriole. DP, deep skin; ART, cut of a subdermal arteriole; HYP, hypodermis; FbE, broken elastic fibre.

Application to the clinical examination of the abdominal wall

Taking these studies into account, a certain number of questions will occur to the plastic surgeon regarding the abdominal wall.

1. What is the state of the elastic network in patients who have a stretchmarked or striated abdomen?

It can be assumed that there will be a very damaged dermal framework, but the real question is, are the anatomicropathological lesions under study really similar to those caused by ageing? In other words, can one talk about a premature ageing of the skin? Remember that the average age of the patients in the authors' study was 31.8 years; among these were six cases of stage I or II lesions, and 13 cases of stage III or IV lesions. The first observation is that there is a contradiction between an average young age (31.8 years) and constant dermal dystrophic lesions, which are often considerable. Among these patients, who are all younger than the crucial age of 45, the lesions are mostly types II, III and IV. This could mean that there is a premature damaging of the dermal elastic tissue. This sample of patients therefore covers a population of subjects with pathological skin.

The skin's appearance is the same as that seen in ageing, and the process seems to have been accelerated. Therefore, we can speak of the premature ageing in the skin of this group of patients (Figs 7.5, 7.6).

2. What preoperative means do we have to assess the elastic capacity of the abdominal wall?

This is of course an essential question for therapeutic strategy, the choice of type of surgery, and the surgical indication. The advent of the technique of liposuction reinforces the importance of this assessment: indeed, liposuction should be followed by a redraping of the skin over the 'new' underlying volumes. If this redraping is deficient, there will be formation of 'waves' or 'corrugated iron'-like skin, which is unaesthetic and unacceptable. In order to avoid this possibility, either such a procedure should not be undertaken or cutaneous reduction plasty with excision and redraping of any skin excess should be carried out as well.

This aspect of preoperative assessment for liposuction is especially important when the abdominal wall is concerned, for the following reasons:

- The thick abdominal skin is not the site of choice for liposuction.

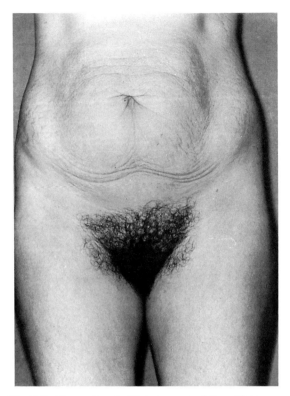

Fig. 7.5 Observation 2: Clinical aspect of the patient, front view.

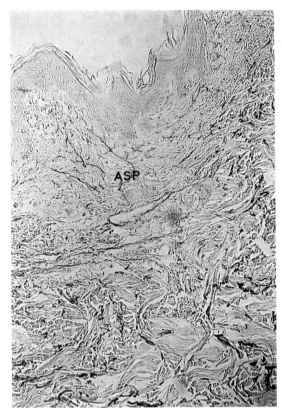

Fig. 7.6 Horizontal section of the skin of the abdomen of patient seen in Fig. 7.5 after color technique with ocein.

• This skin has often been distended by pregnancy, by excess weight or by laparotomy.
• Women are very critical of any irregularity or slight asymmetry in their abdomens.
• Abdominal liposuction is tricky because it is difficult to maintain a regular and symmetrical movement over the whole abdominal wall.

It is therefore very important to be able to judge the capacity of the skin to retract and to redrape itself harmoniously and spontaneously over the underlying structures. Some elements discussed in Chapter 2 should be considered. These are:

(a) The ratio between the amount of excess fat to be sucked out and the area of skin involved. We know that the most favourable case is when the excess fat is moderate, within a limited area. Patients with abundant and diffuse excess fat might face the problem of poor skin retraction capacity.

(b) Date of birth. We have seen that the 45th year seem to be the critical one for dermal and elastic tissue lesions. In practice the physiological age of the underlying skin of the area to be aspirated should be considered.

(c) Cutaneous physiological age. It is important to take this into consideration since the abdominal wall could present early ageing factors. One should consider the thickness of the skin, its tonicity, its extensibility and its elasticity, and look for early local ageing signs such as stretchmarks, folds or dermal atrophy.

(d) The tests. Some tests have been described for liposuction that will enable the evaluation of the spontaneous redraping capacity of the skin. One of these is specific to the abdomen – the test 'for muscular inspection' of Illouz (Fig. 7.7). This resembles the plasticity test of Vilain for the hips, but here the cutaneous laxity is obtained by tensing the anterolateral muscles of the abdomen.

The test consists of inspecting the abdominal wall in the sitting or the upright position, first at rest and then after asking the patient to 'swallow his belly'. This raises the diaphragm and provokes the contraction of the oblique muscles and the transversus abdominis, which pull on the rectus abdominis. When the abdominal wall is intact it follows the movement and leaves no excess. When it has lost its elasticity, a number of folds will appear that reflect the

potential results of an isolated liposuction. By pulling the abdominal skin down to the pubis, the surgeon can assess the height of the excision necessary to return the abdominal wall to normal tension over the underlying volume.

3. Is it possible to form one or several reasonable pathological hypotheses?

From the point of view of the pathogenesis of this premature ageing, several mechanisms can be considered. An analytical study of these is suggested; tissue ageing is a complex phenomenon, not completely understood and probably somewhat variable. Genetic inheritance is a factor to be taken into account. There is clinical evidence of the frequency of certain problems and deformities in the figure in certain families. This

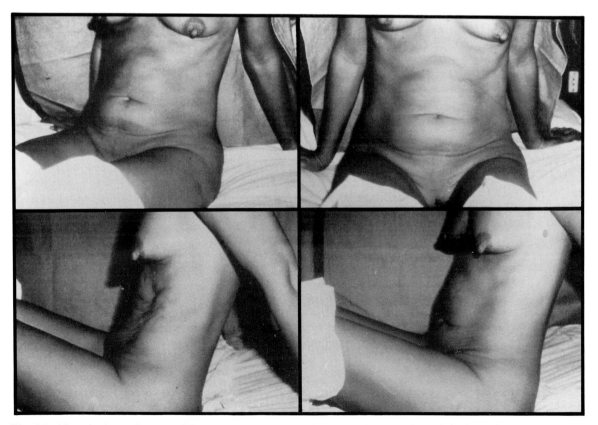

Fig. 7.7 Muscular inspection test of Illouz. Allows evaluation of the retraction capacity and elasticity of the abdominal skin during muscular contraction.

could mean a congenital weakness or dystrophy in elastic tissue and collagen.

A second factor is pregnancy: if pregnancy is multiple and frequent, damage or changes can be seen in the abdomen and breasts of many women. Mechanical stress is often given as the cause, but this is not sufficient. Hormonal saturation during gestation acts on the skin, collagen, elastic fibres and adipose tissue. According to Robert, 'it is a cliché to say that. . . under the same physical conditions, with equivalent skins, different hormonal environments will lead to different lesions'.

Lipid metabolism involves an interaction between the metabolic and the mechanical factors, and their influence on elastic fibres. We have seen how lipophilic protein can electively fix lipids as well as calcium: this double fixation and the complexity it brings about in the fibres causes a loss of elasticity and, therefore, a weakening of the molecule. It is easy to understand, and Jacotot and Robert explain that a fibre which has lost its elasticity but remains subject to the same mechanical demands is going to break down.

The mechanical factors are closely linked to the metabolic and hormonal factors; the main ones are pregnancy and obesity. At the cellular level the excess weight causes a dilatation of the subdermal fatty cells which are overflowing with adipocytes. The deep fibrous spans which separate the compartments of adipose tissue are distended. Moreover, their elastic framework is progressively weakened by calcium and lipid fixation. If the weight gain continues, the fibrous spans, having lost all their elasticity, will break under the excess weight of the adipose lobules. If there is a rapid, marked weight loss, there is no way to prevent the sagging of the abdominal skin, the skin of the breasts and buttocks, and the inner portion of the arm: this is unavoidable. The skin has lost its elasticity and its tone; stretchmarks appear as a sign of disruption of elasticity. This disruption, for biomechanical reasons, is often seen in the abdominal wall.

Massive weight gain followed by quick weight-loss diets is extremely dangerous.

4. Is it possible to give a prognosis of the various conditions, and then to speak of their prevention and therapy?

Prevention has been described in detail in Chapter 3. As far as therapy is concerned, surgical possibilities depend greatly on the quality of the residual skin and on what will be required of it.

It is interesting to observe that lesions of the abdominal wall do not affect the median and deep skin. This is a good omen for a successful surgery, theoretically better than lesions involving the breast, for example. It is valid, therefore, to rely on good quality residual skin during reconstruction of the abdominal wall. If a large excision is performed the mechanical pull should be reduced as much as possible.

8. Operative techniques

In the years since the previous edition of this book, operative techniques have progressed dramatically. This chapter will deal with this progress and its two main modalities. Truly new techniques have emerged, such as liposuction; this could well be a therapeutic treatment by itself, or a complementary step in an otherwise classic abdominoplasty. There have also been technical modifications to existing procedures; these are surgical refinements that increase the efficiency and refine the results of classic operations. This is the case, for example, in surgical procedures to minimize the residual scar, to cosmetically improve the umbilical area, or to perfect the tension of the musculoaponeurotic layer.

CLASSIC TECHNIQUES

There are many operative techniques, whose number reflects the obvious difficulty encountered in the search for perfection. They are generally described as abdominoplasties, and deal with different indications and try to correct different conditions. Since the end of the last century there have been periodic descriptions of new techniques, until about 1960. Since then the literature has greatly increased. However, classification by the type of incision has not changed since Corréa Iturraspe in 1952, who described three groups: transverse incisions, generally inferiorly located, among which must be distinguished anterior abdominoplasties, three-quarter abdominoplasties and circular abdominoplasties; vertical or longitudinal incisions: generally median and occasionally lateral; and combined incisions associating the previous two types.

This classification will be respected throughout this study. For historical purposes, the name of the author and year of publication will be indicated for each main type of operation. The most commonly used techniques will then be described in detail. Whenever possible, the drawings of the author himself will be used, thus helping the reader to distinguish one procedure from another.

Horizontal or transverse abdominoplasty

This category includes all types of horizontal incision at right-angles to the xiphopubic line, regardless of their relationship to the umbilicus. Such incisions tend to stretch more or less laterally for the optimum result in a circular lipectomy. These operations aim to pull down the abdomen. This can be achieved by:

- Pulling strictly from top to bottom, creating two 'dog-ears' which may call for a final correction.
- Pulling downwards and inwards in the 'setting-sun' manner of Vilain, with a transverse excess of skin causing folds that will take a long time to disappear.
- Pulling downwards and outwards, after the technique of Pitanguy, in which case the skin is much better draped although the length of the scar is drawn laterally.

As early as 1890, Demars and Marx achieved the first resection of an abdominal apron through an 'orange' segment — a subumbilical incision.

Kelly, in 1899 (Fig. 8.1), introduced the term 'lipectomy', and used a transverse half-moon incision over the umbilicus, which was sacrificed in the process.

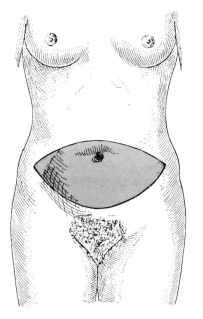 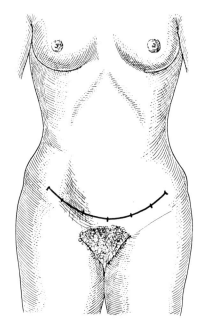

Fig. 8.1   Kelly (1899), Morestin (1912).

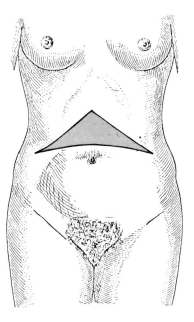 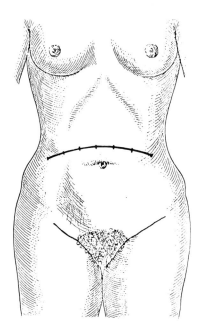

Fig. 8.2   Thorek (1923).

Schutz, Schallenberg and Jolly in 1911 used the technique of Kelly, adapting it for the correction of an umbilical hernia.

Morestin in his thesis in 1912 gives recognition to the process of Kelly.

Thorek (Fig. 8.2), in 1923, described his own

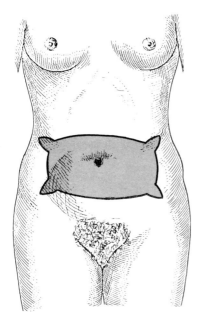

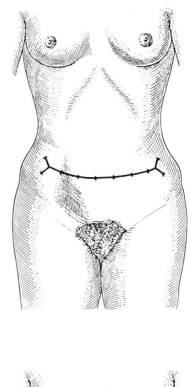

Fig. 8.3   Delbet (1928).

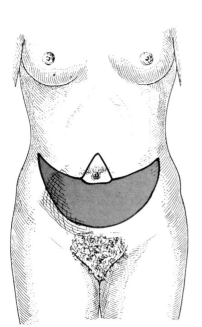

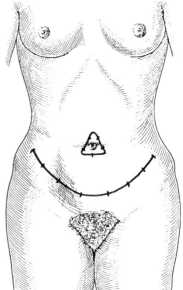

Fig. 8.4   Flesh, Thebesius (1931).

technique for abdominoplasty, which helps to remodel the breast at the same time. He carried out resection and traction at the supraumbilical level through a subcostal incision shaped like a batwing.

Delbert (Fig. 8.3), in 1928, did a horizontal

rectangular resection centred on the umbilicus, and corrected the lateral ears through a Y-shaped suture.

Flesh, Thebesius and Wheishemer (Fig. 8.4), in 1931, performed the first umbilical transposition but transposed an equilateral triangle of skin centred on the umbilicus.

Mornard (Fig. 8.5), in 1938, accomplished the first true umbilical transposition.

Vernon (Fig. 8.6), in 1957, in the United States described a perfectly regulated technique of subumbilical plasty with transposition of the umbilicus. The lateral flaps were corrected through two triangular resections, ending in two small descending vertical scars at either end of the incision.

Dufourmentel and Mouly in (Fig. 8.7), in their treaty on plastic surgery in 1959, as well as Morel-Fatio in the Voloir thesis of 1960, described the technique of low transverse anterior lipectomy, which is now a classic and is still popularly used: the inferior line, drawn with the patient standing, follows the upper border of the pubic hair, slanting laterally in the inguinal folds toward the anterior iliac spine. The superior line, drawn by holding the subumbilical excess of fatty tissue in both hands, reunites the two extremities of the above line, but is only temporary. The umbilicus is incised several millimetres from its periphery. The upper flap is then detached in the direction of the xiphoid and the costal margin. The resection of the skin and fat depends on how far the flap can be pulled downwards (Fig. 8.8).

There are many variations of this subumbilical anterior abdominal lipectomy with transposition of the umbilicus. Some will be described while others are merely mentioned.

Pitanguy (Figs 8.9–8.11), published another method which he used on 300 patients. This uses a low transverse incision without a midline resection; the inferior incision extends horizontally on either side of the pubic triangle and curves bilaterally downwards and outwards at the intersection of the inguinal fold, which it crosses, and then goes horizontally up to the apex of the anterior superior iliac spine, and finally curves slightly downwards.

Callia's (1965) technique (Figs 8.12–8.14) draws the lateral parts of the incision 2 cm beneath the inguinal folds, lower than Pitanguy's. To facilitate the dissection, the superior flap is divided into two inferior abdominal flaps, the in-

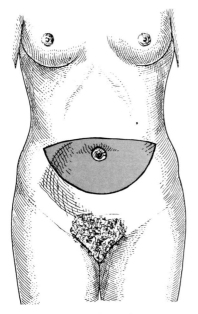
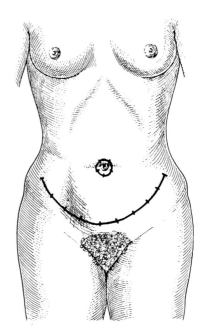

Fig. 8.5 Mornard (1938).

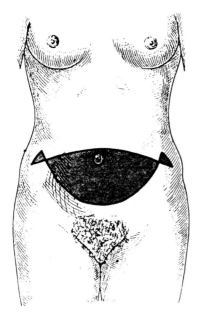 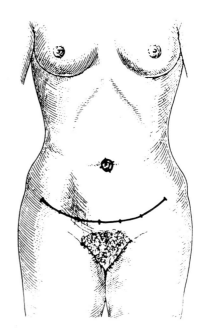

Fig. 8.6 Vernon (1957).

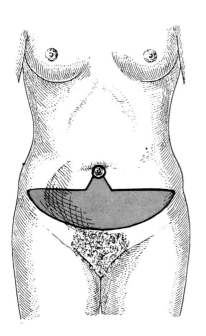 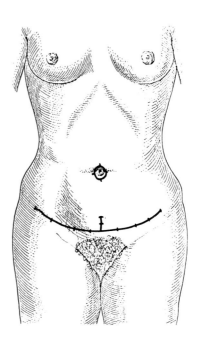

Fig. 8.7 Dufourmentel, Mouly (1959).

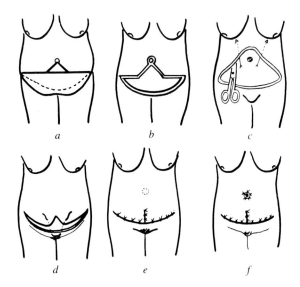

Fig. 8.8 Technique of abdominal plasty with transposition of the umbilicus (From C. Dufourmentel and R. Mouly).

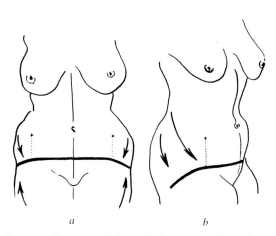

Fig. 8.9 Transverse abdominal plasty, a technique of Pitanguy. Front and lateral view (**a** and **b**), show the horizontal incisions that curves downward when it reaches the vertical projection of the anterior superior iliac spine.

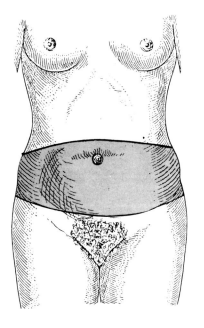

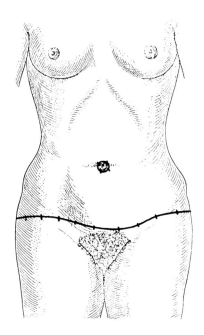

Fig. 8.10 Pitanguy (1967).

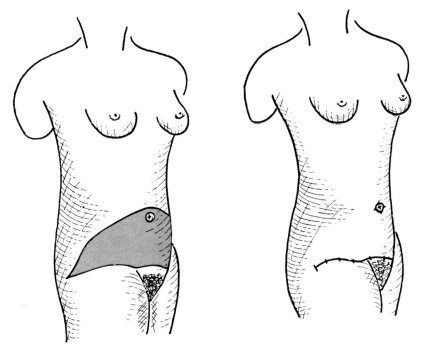

Fig. 8.11 Pitanguy (1967).

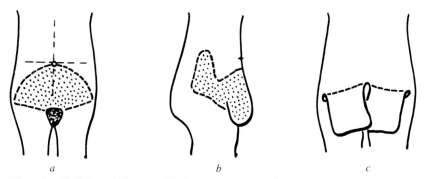

a   *b*   *c*

Fig. 8.12 Callia's technique modified by Lagache and Vandenbusche. **a** The incision lines, front view. **b** This sketch characterizes the lateral modification which was brought to the original Callia technique by the author. **c** Detail technique emphasizing the importance of bringing together the bilateral abdominal flaps after their resection in order to avoid the lateral dogears.

cision being in the midline. He then pulls the highest point of the abdominal flap down over the pubis; this permits the resection of the two quadrangular flaps.

Vandenbusche (Figs 8.15, 8.16), in 1971, modified Callia's procedure by adding a stepwise resection on either side, proceeding laterally and upwards on the transverse incision. This permits a better longitudinal draping of the skin.

Grazer, in 1973, added a modification to the technique of Pitanguy.

D. Serson Neto (Fig. 8.17), in 1959, proposed a geometrical approach to abdominoplasty with his 'decagon' technique. The sketch of the

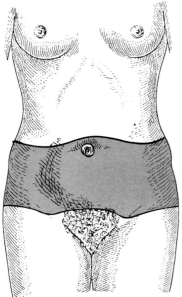
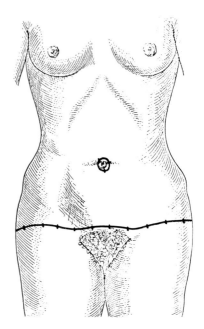

Fig. 8.13 Callia (1967).

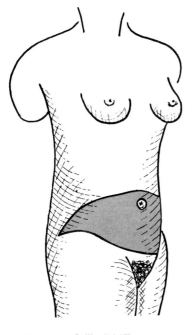
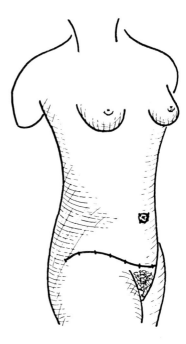

Fig. 8.14 Callia (1967).

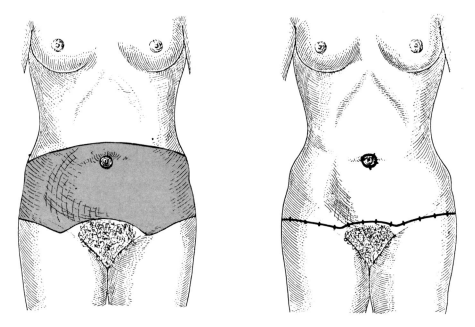

Fig. 8.15 Callia modified by Lagache and Vandenbusche (1971).

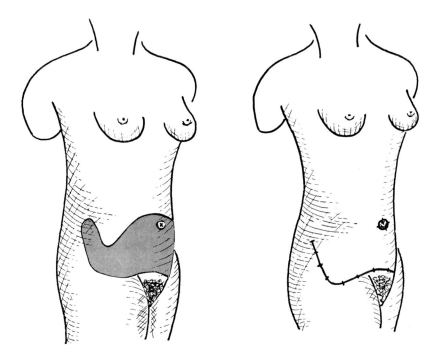

Fig. 8.16 Callia modified by Lagache and Vandenbusche (1971).

incision is well codified, leaving no doubt as to interpretation. Surgery can be shortened because of the limited detachment. The differences in the length of the incision edges are also reduced (Fig. 8.17).

Baroudi (Figs 8.18, 8.19), in 1974, described his own technique: the lower incision line resembles a wide-angled 'W', with a middle part going over the pubic hair and with the lateral ends crossing over the inguinal folds by 1–3 cm.

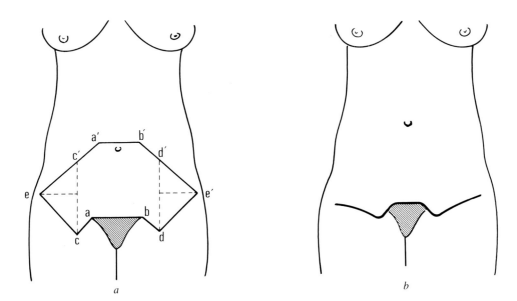

Fig. 8.17 'Decagon' technique. (D. Serson Neto, 1969). **a** incisions; **b** scar line.

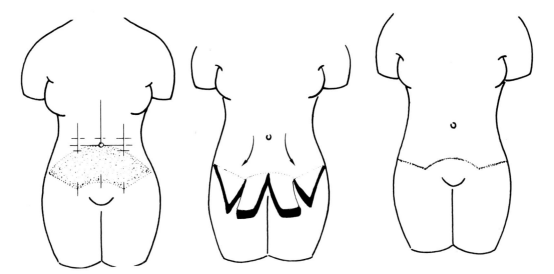

Fig. 8.18 Technique used to determine the portion of skin which has to be resected to avoid any asymmetry of the incision. (R. Baroudi, P. R. S., 1974, p. 54, Williams & Wilkins, Baltimore)

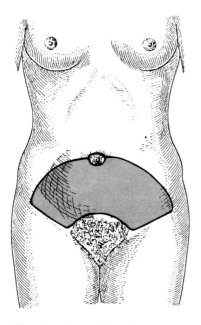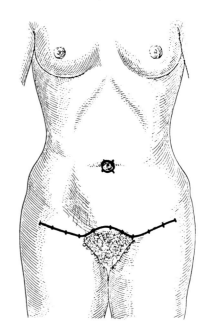

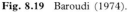

Fig. 8.19 Baroudi (1974).

The detached area forms a triangle whose superior angle faces the xiphoid and whose base corresponds to the inferior incision line which has been described. The superior border of the resection is determined, as in the technique of Callia, by pulling down the superior abdominal flap. The author particularly stresses the care which must be given to the area around the umbilicus in order to maintain its natural appearance. To do this, a small transverse incision must first be made on the skin of the superior flap at the projection of the umbilicus. The undersurface of the superior flap is then defatted. Four nylon sutures are placed through the skin of the abdominal wall, the rectus sheath and the skin edges of the umbilicus, as shown in Fig. 8.20. When the knots are tied, the edges of the abdominal skin incision curve naturally toward the umbilicus. Finally, in case of weakness or diastasis recti, the author suggests an overlapping of the two aponeurotic edges, while making a small transverse incision in each one to achieve a correctly placed suture.

Paule Regnault (Fig. 8.21), in 1975, also suggested a lower W-shaped incision with a median triangle, the upper part of which would be in the area of the pubic hair, and the lower lateral branches in the inguinal folds (Fig. 8.22).

Vilain (Fig. 8.23), in 1975, published the 'setting sun' technique.

CIRCULAR LIPECTOMY

Described by González Ulloa (Figs 8.24, 8.25) in 1960, introduced in France and modified by Vilain in 1964 (Figs 8.26, 8.27), this technique excises a large fatty-cutaneous circumferential

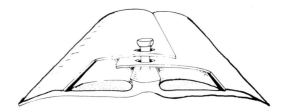

Fig. 8.20 Suturing the umbilicus. This diagram shows the major muscles and the white umbilical line, hidden by the upper abdominal flap. Each suture anchors at the same time the abdominal skin, the aponeurosis, and the skin of the abdominal flap. (R. Baroudi, Plast Reconstr Surg 1974, p. 54, Williams & Wilkins, Baltimore)

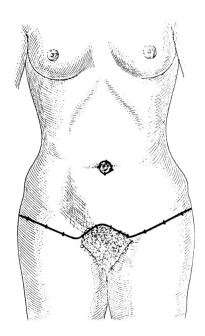

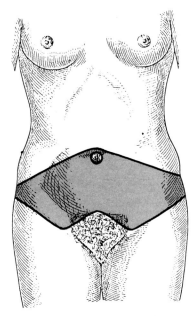

Fig. 8.21 P. Regnault (1975).

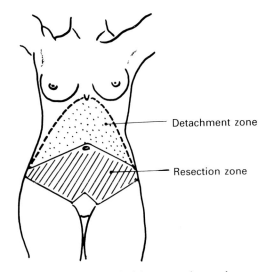

Detachment zone

Resection zone

Fig. 8.22 Sketch of the incisions, resection, and detachment in the 'W' technique (P. Regnault)

cylinder of skin from the abdomen (Fig. 8.28). This is a major and difficult operation. It cannot be seen as cosmetic, as there are many resulting scars, but some results seen after 15–20 years are remarkable. In the authors' opinion, however, it is meant only for abdomens marred by enormous and irreversible forms of obesity, which seem to be increasingly rare. Nowadays, these patients could benefit from abdominal liposuction extended laterally to the sides and to the lumbar area. Consequently, the rare patient that 10 years ago would have needed a circular lipectomy, would today benefit from a classic low transverse abdominoplasty associated with liposuction of the sides and the lumbar area.

VERTICAL OR LONGITUDINAL ABDOMINOPLASTY

This section will describe all the techniques based on axial resection following the xiphopubic line.

Apart from the direction of the incision, these techniques differ from the preceding ones in their indications. If the transverse lipectomy is the operation of choice for the obese, vertical resection is intended mostly for the woman whose abdomen after pregnancy has become wrinkled, creased or marred by excess skin. The illustrations show better than any text the evolution of these techniques: Spaulding, 1901 (Fig. 8.29), Babcock, 1916, Schepelman, 1918 (Fig. 8.30), Kuster, 1926.

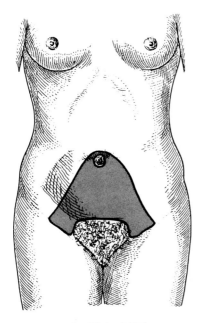
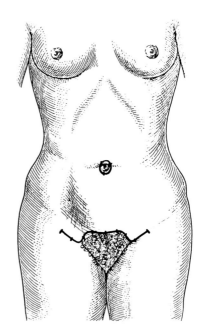

Fig. 8.23   R. Vilain (1975).

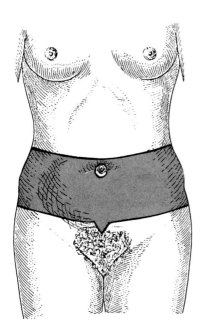
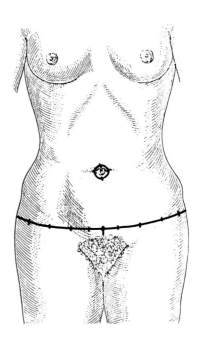

Fig. 8.24   M. G. Ulloa (1960).

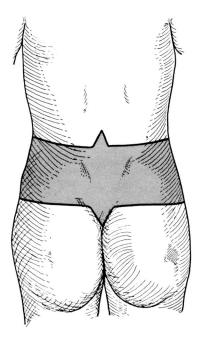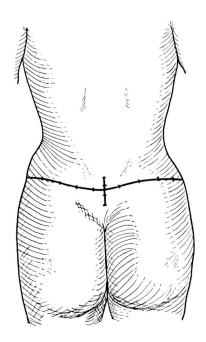

Fig. 8.25 M. G. Ulloa (1960).

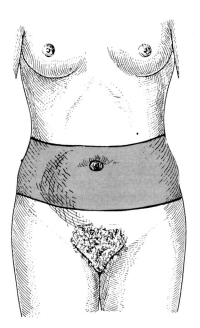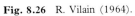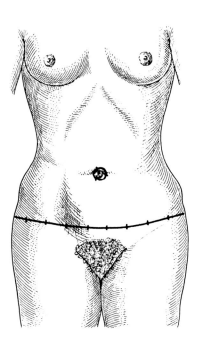

Fig. 8.26 R. Vilain (1964).

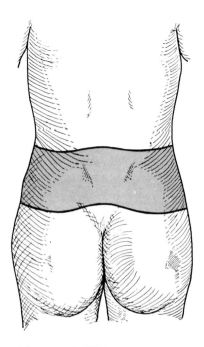 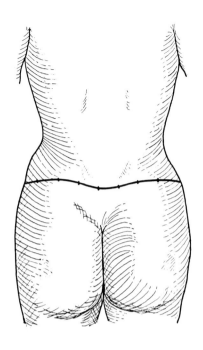

Fig. 8.27 R. Vilain (1964).

Marchal and Lapeyrie, in 1964, described a biconvex vertical resection whose upper and lower lines end in a 'fish tail' arrangement. The skin approximation at the end of the operation is above and below the umbilicus, with a Y-shaped incision at either end. Among this large series of vertical abdominoplasties, the most simple technique, and also the one most often performed, is that of Fischl (1973; Figs 8.31, 8.32). A large ellipse of medial vertical skin is excised, from one end of the abdomen to the other. The part to be resected is assessed by approximation with both hands. A triangle is made at either end of the incision to avoid 'dog ears'. The umbilicus, which was initially circumscribed, reappears at its proper place in the midline scar at the end of the operation.

In the same year, Picaud proposed a midline vertical fusiform resection, using the idea of vertical abdominoplasty for correction of certain deformities; especially for women with an excess of unattractive periumbilical skin.

To summarize, a vertical excision has two advantages: it is better when the excess skin has a longer vertical diameter than horizontal; it also brings the lateral skin toward the centre and decreases the size of the waist. Such an operation, which is far from ideal, may be the only possible option for long, stretchmarked and wrinkled abdomens.

COMBINED DERMOLIPECTOMY

Combined dermolipectomy is useful in principle because it allows resection and even a reduction both horizontally and vertically, which is ideal when trying to remove an excess of skin. However, in practice there are two major disadvantages:

1. There are prominent scars, in the shape of an anchor, that are unattractive.
2. There is a positive risk of necrosis at the weakest point, where the three flaps are sutured together.

Most surgeons prefer transverse incisions, some of which have small vertical resections, which are in fact combined incisions. Rockay, in 1893,

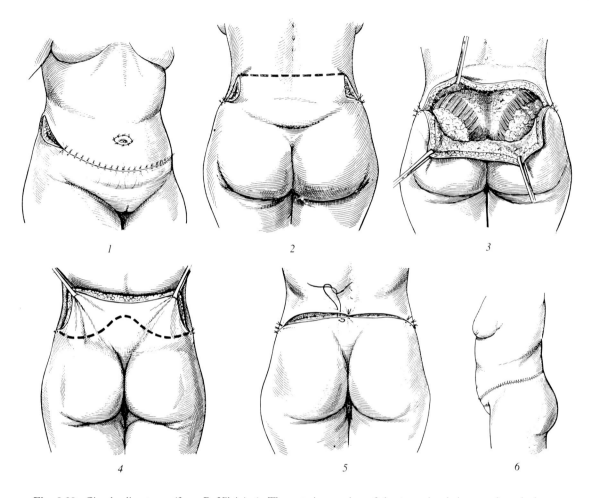

Fig. 8.28 Circular lipectomy (from R. Vilain). 1. The anterior portion of the operation being terminated, the lateral ends of the incision must be left open. 2. The posterior incision; a horizontal line rejoins the upper end of the incision. 3. Posterior undermining is not brought up very far superiorly. It can go quite low behind, even to include a defatting of the buttocks. Vilain recommends not undermining too far down in the back to avoid interference with the lymphatics. 4. A scalloped line is the only modification brought by Vilain to the original technique of M. G. Ulloa. It allows an excellent conformity of the two flaps and helps to form a normal-looking waist. 5. Posterior suturing. 6. Profile view.

described the first three-branch incision, giving an inverted T-shaped scar below the umbilicus (Fig. 8.33).

Weinhold, in 1913, achieved three elliptical incisions converging in the subumbilical area; the umbilicus remains in place. The scar has the shape of a three-sided helix (Fig. 8.34).

Galtier, in 1955, associated a horizontal and a vertical resection which were perfectly perpendicular and intersected at the umbilicus. The technique is well codified and the markings are very precise (Fig. 8.35). The results are often quite satisfactory with regard to tightening the abdomen and decreasing the size of the waist, but the scar is most unsightly.

Barraya, in 1967, taking into account the lines of tension of the abdominal wall, drew a dermolipectomy in the form of a crossbow. The two inferior horizontal curvilinear incisions go along the superior border of the pubis and the inguinal folds. The two vertical median markings meet superiorly after bypassing the umbilicus, which will be reconstructed (Fig. 8.36).

Thomeret, in 1971, after studying the disad-

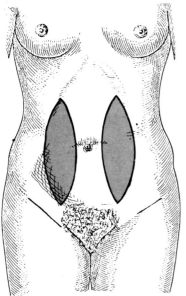
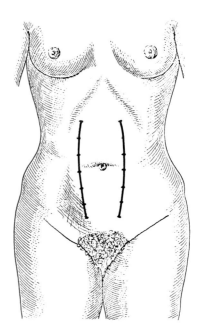

Fig. 8.29 Spaulding (1901).

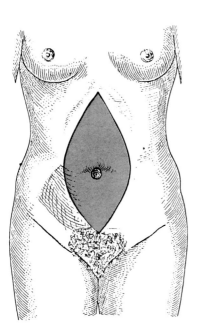
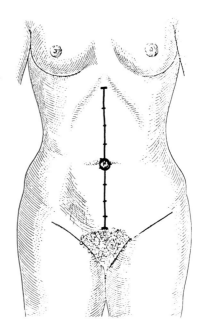

Fig. 8.30 Schepelman (1918).

vantages of the combined techniques and the circular lipectomies of González Ulloa and Vilain, which do not decrease the waist sufficiently, described an operation which is a combination of these techniques. The extent of the necessary anterior resection can be visualized by gathering the abdominal skin together with both hands. The midline vertical resection ends in a point at the xiphoid and at the pubis. The horizontal resection extends in a circle into the back.

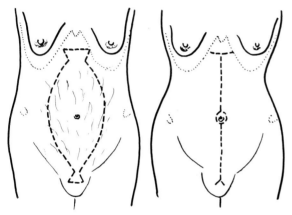

Fig. 8.31 Vertical abdominoplasty, showing lines of incisions and suture lines (from R. A. Fischl).

MORE RECENT TECHNIQUES

This section concerns techniques, not all of them new, that adapt the surgical procedure to the different lesions, resulting in simpler operations and smaller scars.

Localized abdominoplasty

These are for limited lesions. The principle behind them is to adapt a cutaneous reduction plasty to a lesion, resulting in a smaller resection and substituting small scars for large and, if possible, concealed ones. Their definition is anatomical and will depend on the area of the lesion and the incision. There are three types: plasties of the subumbilical area, plasties of the midabdomen and of the periumbilical area, and plasties of the supraumbilical area. Procedures to improve the scar will also be discussed.

Subumbilical abdominoplasty: the 'horseshoe' technique (Elbaz 1974, Figs 8.37, 8.38)

The principle here is to resect a portion of skin and fat around the pubic triangle, in the shape

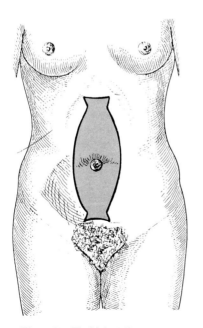
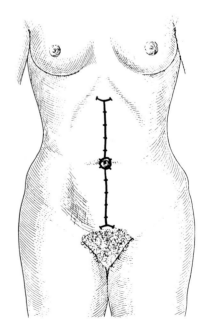

Fig. 8.32 Fischl (1973).

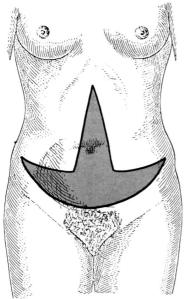

Fig. 8.33 Rockay (1893).

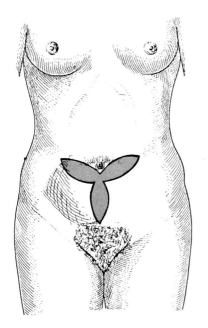

Fig. 8.34 Weinhold (1913).

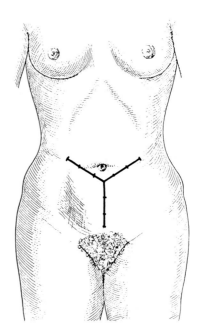

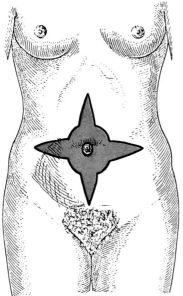
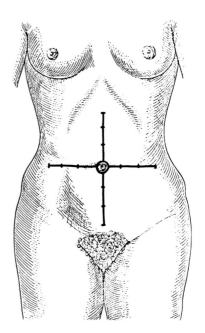

Fig. 8.35   Galtier (1955).

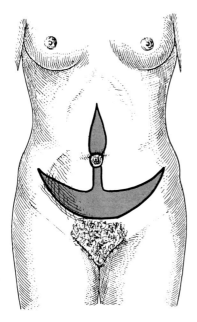
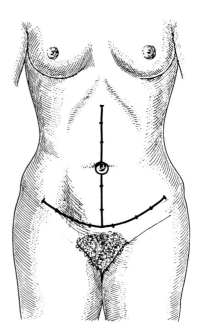

Fig. 8.36   Barraya (1967).

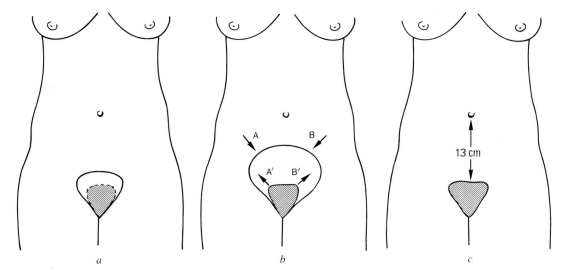

Fig. 8.37 The 'horse shoe' technique. (J. S. Elbaz, 1974.)

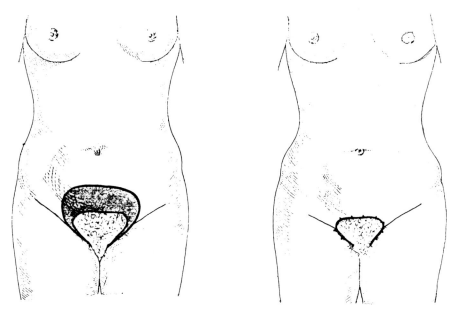

Fig. 8.38 J. S. Elbaz (1974).

of a horseshoe. The incision is in the pubic hair and follows its upper border, with a midline superior convex portion and two lateral portions curving downwards and inwards toward the genitocrural area. The peripheral line of the incision resembles a horseshoe, and two skin advancements at points A and B must be left to reduce the tension. The undermining is carried out superiorly until the fatty-cutaneous wall can be advanced over the pubis. There is no transposition of the umbilicus.

Two thick sutures fix points A and A' and B and B'. The skin closure starts with the transverse section AB. The incongruity is easy to correct.

There will be a dog ear at either end of the suture, which will be hidden since it is located in the perineum.

Beside the release of tension in the inferior abdominal flap, this operation helps to remove the major portion of an appendectomy or subumbili-cal scar, if they are present. The spreading of the pubic triangle due to traction returns it to an almost normal size.

The indications should be carefully considered. The main advantage is in the resulting small and concealed scar.

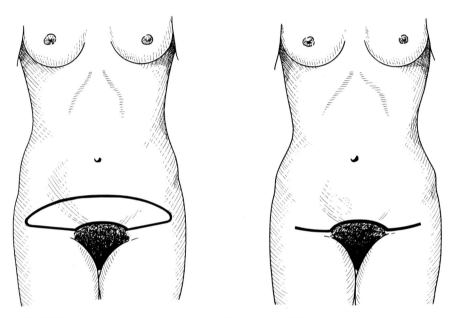

Fig. 8.39 Low transverse abdominoplasty without any umbilical procedure.

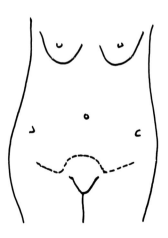

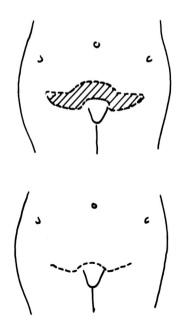

Fig. 8.40 Minilift for excess of skin in the area of the lower abdomen (Glicenstein, modified by Serson); sketch of the resected area, the area of the scar (a simple suprapubic incision is sufficient).

Low transverse abdominoplasty without umbilical procedure

If the lesion, despite being subumbilical, does not allow a 'horseshoe' technique, a low transverse abdominoplasty without umbilical transposition can be considered.

If there is excess skin in the subumbilical area, with low lesions such as stretchmarks or scars, a low, crescent-shaped transverse abdominoplasty can be performed if the rest of the abdominal wall is in good condition (Fig. 8.39). In this operation, nothing is done to the umbilicus: neither an umbilical transposition nor an umbilical disinsertion will be carried out. This strategy results in an increase in distance between the umbilicus and the pubic triangle.

This type of operation was published by Glicenstein in 1975, and was known as 'abdominal minilifting' (Figs 8.40–8.42). It has subsequently been called 'limited abdominoplasty' (Wilkinson et al. 1986) and 'miniabdominoplasty' (Greminger 1987).

Technically, the distance between the umbilicus and the pubis is measured first with the skin tensed and then with the skin loose. The difference between the two measurements gives the height of the skin to be resected (1–1.5 cm could easily be added). The excision circumscribes the pubis lateral and goes upwards in the inguinal folds. After excision, an upward detachment is carried out, level with the aponeurosis as far as the umbilicus and a little higher on each side. It should be easy to approximate the superior flap without deforming the umbilicus.

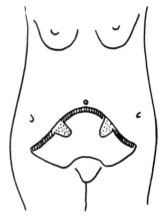

Fig. 8.41 Two strips of skin are peeled off which will be planted under the skin of the pubic area (Glicenstein, modified by Serson). In Annales de Chirurgie Plastique, 1975, Vol. XX, No. 2.

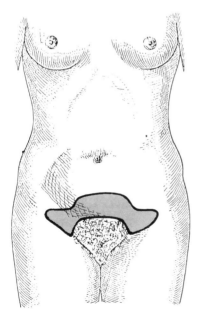
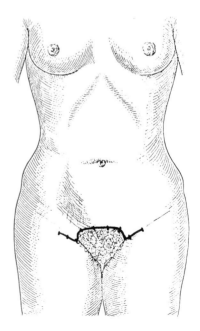

Fig. 8.42 J. Glicenstein (1975).

This type of operation, associated with liposuction and the use of a biological glue, will be described in Chapter 10.

Compared to the horseshoe this transverse incision allows an easier correction of the 'ears' laterally in the inguinal folds, but the scars are more obvious. However, if the approximation of the superior flap causes a distortion of the umbilicus, an umbilical disinsertion must be performed, with a lowering of the umbilicus.

Low transverse abdominoplasty with umbilical disinsertion

Most of the difficulties with abdominoplasty are due to the umbilicus and to the 'mooring' between the skin and the aponeurosis and muscles at this level. For almost a century, the tightening of the abdominal skin was held back by the question of whether or not to carry out an umbilical transposition, and whether the supraumbilical skin could be lowered to the pubic area without distending and raising the pubic triangle.

Callia, in 1975 described umbilical disinsertion, freeing surgeons from the above questions and opening the way to new therapeutic possibilities, especially in the case of post pregnancy dermal dystrophies (Fig. 8.43). This same idea was presented by Guimberteau and Goin in 1983, and by Thion in 1985. It is thus important that the umbilicus should no longer be seen as an obstacle to reshaping the abdominal wall.

There are a number of indications for umbilical disinsertion.

1. Excess skin in the subumbilical area in a low transverse abdominoplasty, when the lowering of the upper flap is difficult and distorts the umbilicus.
2. Moderate skin excess in the supraumbilical and periumbilical area.
3. Umbilical disinsertion permits the tightening of moderately distended supraumbilical and periumbilical areas without leaving a periumbilical scar. Technically, it results in the lowering of the umbilicus. This is acceptable (a) because even though the distance between the umbilicus and the pubic triangle is almost always the same (approximately 13 cm), it could be reduced to 11 or even 10 cm without altering the aesthetic equilibrium of the abdomen, and (b) because the lower edge of the incision is

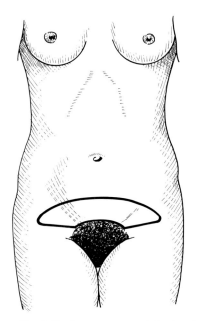
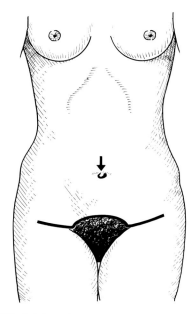

Fig. 8.43 Low transverse abdominoplasty with umbilical disinsertion.

2–3 cm below the upper side of the pubic triangle, which itself is therefore 2–3 cm lower. For these two reasons, the umbilicus could be lowered by 2–3 cm.

Technique

The incision of the lower edge is 2–3 cm below the upper edge of the pubic triangle, and proceeds laterally into the inguinal folds, depending on the size of the skin resection. The detachment extends upward as necessary, without restriction, because of the umbilical disinsertion. The umbilicus is sectioned level with the aponeurosis. The resulting aponeurotic hole is closed off with strong buried sutures. The umbilicus, together with the abdominal skin, is lowered by cutaneous redraping as necessary. At least 10 cm should separate the umbilicus and the pubic triangle (Fig. 8.44a,b,c,d).

The umbilicus is then implanted and attached by two sutures to the aponeurosis exactly at the midline. It will retain its normal morphology, with no scar.

This method facilitates the treatment of subumbilical, supraumbilical and periumbilical malformations, leaving no scar on the hairless skin.

Umbilical disinsertion eases the tension from the pubic scar, preventing it from rising or becoming wider. Furthermore this scar is located low down, and could be easily hidden by underwear.

Umbilical disinsertion is not the solution to every problem; it is acceptable only if the redraping is done by lowering the skin approximately 2–3 cm, as described above.

Liposuction and an aponeurotic muscular plasty could be carried out at the same time.

Plasties of the midabdomen and periumbilical area

Strictly umbilical and periumbilical lesions cannot be corrected from a distant incision such as the one described. These represent one of the major difficulties of abdominoplasty. The choice remains between downwards tension, which is always possible, and a direct approach to the lesion with a midabdominal scar. The patient must already have been warned about the exact location of the future scar, its size and its prognosis. Three possible scenarios will be described; the indications are very few and the patient must give fully informed consent.

Periumbilical circular plasty

This consists of a circular excision forming a periumbilical disk, but this operation is not recommended because either the excision is too small, or, if big enough, the following three phenomena may result:

1. 'Sunray pleats' that do not always disappear.
2. The umbilicus does not remain at the bottom of its crater and becomes larger.
3. The scar is often visible because of its exteriorization, and is often hypertrophic because of the skin tension that acts on it (Fig. 8.45).

Transverse supraumbilical abdominoplasty

This technique was proposed by Vilain, mainly for stretchmarked, crinkled and creased supraumbilical areas. Its originality stems from the fact that it could be performed under local anesthetic in two or three separate procedures, allowing maximum advantage to be taken of the skin elasticity, and reducing the final scar.

The procedure consists of a short horizontal transverse supraumbilical fusiform excision. After a prudent first excision, without trying to 'absorb' all the skin excess, a second excision is performed a few months later, from the first scar. The upper edge is detached upwards in order to allow a complementary excision of the residual skin without extending the scar. The result will be a short horizontal midabdominal scar located directly above the umbilicus; its middle portion can be partially concealed in the umbilical crater (Fig. 8.46).

Midabdominoplasty

This is designed for lesions localized around the umbilicus, but too spread out and extensive for the two techniques described above. It consists

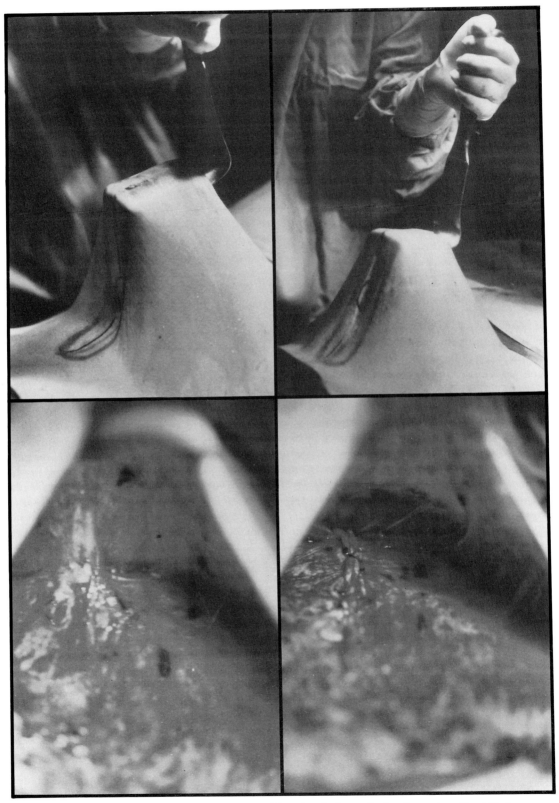

Fig. 8.44 a, b, c, d Per-operative views of umbilical disinsertion, before and after the section of umbilical attachments.

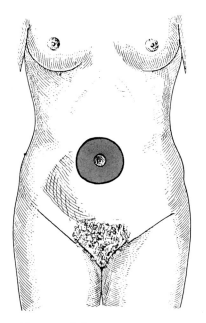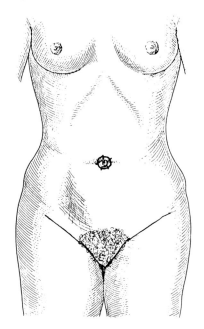

Fig. 8.45 J. S. Elbaz (for exceptions, see text).

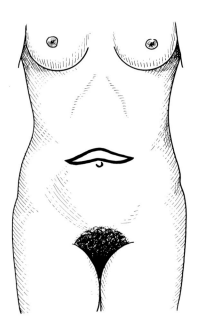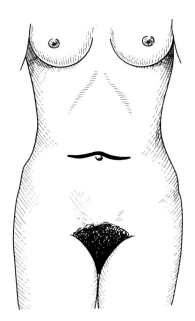

Fig. 8.46 Transverse supraumbilical abdominoplasty.

of a fusiform or elliptical excision with a long horizontal transverse axis centred on the umbilicus. The length and width of the excision depend on the lesion concerned, and determine the size of the resulting scar. The umbilicus will be neither disinserted nor transposed in relation to the parietal abdominal wall, but will remain in its original place.

The technique has not been named and does not correspond to any of the classic ones, although it has been used a good deal with interesting results. Stuckey in 1975 called it the 'midabdomen abdominoplasty'.

Surgery begins with a circular incision and dissection of the umbilicus. Starting from this point, the skin is then detached upwards, downwards and laterally. The excess skin is then easily seen and resected symmetrically upwards and downwards, either elliptically or fusiform. The upper and lower edges are then approximated, resulting in a horizontal midabdominal suture interrupted in its midpoint by the umbilicus.

Two diametrically opposed half-circles, equal in size to the umbilicus, are then excised at the middle of the incision, where the umbilicus will be placed. This technique entirely removes all moderate periumbilical lesions, but has the disadvantage of leaving a large scar in the middle of the abdomen. However, this becomes acceptable after a short period of time.

Plasties of the supraumbilical area: high transverse dermolipectomies

In 1977, Rebello described a technique that is satisfactory for some very precise and rare indications: lesions of the upper abdomen, with no lesions in the subumbilical area (Fig. 8.47).

In its upper part the incision extends laterally, following the inframammary line, and describes in its median and sternal section a downward-oriented concavity, giving it the shape of a gullswing. The supraaponeurotic detachment continues as far as the umbilicus and beyond laterally. The extension of the excision will be evaluated during surgery, by performing an incision on the abdominal flap at its midline and placing a staystitch at the point of maximum traction. In this way the lower edge of the incision will form a curve with an upward concavity, that will meet the inner ends of the inframammary lines. There is no umbilical transposition. A good tightening of the entire supraumbilical skin can be achieved.

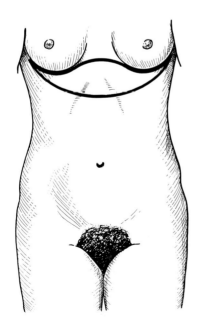
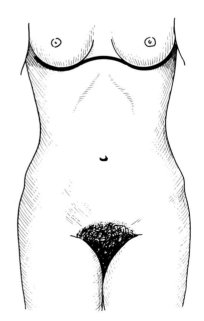

Fig. 8.47 High transverse dermolipectomy.

The main disadvantage of this technique is that it leaves a median transverse sternal scar, bridging between the two breasts. In this area the scars are usually hypertrophic because of the strong local traction forces. One should not be tempted to make large resections in order to reduce these tensional forces. It is also important that the median section of the scar be located low enough to be concealed beneath the brassiere.

The ideal indication for this technique would be the woman presenting with a supraumbilical fatty-cutaneous excess and needing a mammoplasty; in this case the scars would then join.

It should be added that the authors have not noticed any negative effect from this technique on mammary stability. A good detachment eliminates any skin tension and helps prevent this kind of complication.

METHODS OF IMPROVING THE SCAR

Two frequent criticisms of abdominoplasty, concern the tendency of the scar to become invaginated and buried, or to become asymmetrical both in length and height. The following are two methods that have been proposed to prevent such defects.

Invaginated or buried scars

The invagination of a scar is due to its adhesion to the underlying aponeurosis and muscles. Such a scar could end up being buried, a not uncommon complication.

Vilain proposed leaving two fatty-cutaneous deepithelialized triangular flaps, one at each edge of the incision, that will cross at the approximation of the edges and form a 'dermal basement' for the sutured edges, preventing their retraction towards the underlying area.

In the case of a low transverse abdominoplasty with umbilical transposition, a large equilateral fatty-cutaneous triangle should be left each side measuring 6–7 cm, with a pubic base. This triangle will work as a fatty basement for the portion of the superior flap initially located over the umbilicus (see Fig. 8.48).

Asymmetrical scars

A retrospective study of 300 abdominoplasties performed by the authors in 1976, showed how frequently the scar was imperfect in either length and height, or the persistence of an irregular

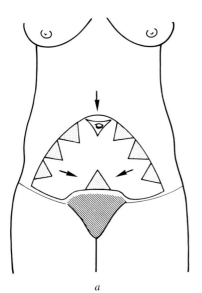
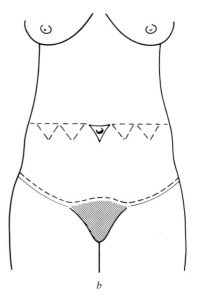

a   *b*

Fig. 8.48   Fatty cutaneous epithelialized triangular flaps, 'the teeth of the sea'. (R. Vilain).

wrinkling of the skin. After this analysis, the following strategy was proposed in order to correct such defects:

1. The incision is drawn symmetrically with the patient standing.
2. After excision and detachment, a staystitch is placed exactly on the midline.
3. From the inside to the outside on each side of the midline, and at 5 cm intervals, the upper edge is approximated by a staystitch and sutured to the lower edge with maximum 'trickery' and minimum puckering of the skin.
4. Symmetry is achieved by transferring the exact value of the 'trickery' on the opposite lower edge for every 5 cm interval measured on the upper edge.

In this way the incongruity of the edges is corrected regularly and symmetrically to the best of skin tolerance (Figs 8.49–8.58).

ABDOMINOPLASTY AND LIPOSUCTION

The different applications of liposuction will be thoroughly explained in Chapter 9. This section will simply examine the main modalities for the association of liposuction with classic dermolipectomy.

It has already been seen that the abdominal wall is an elective site for fat deposition, which has always been a major problem for the surgeon in abdominoplasty. Surgery has never completely taken into account the treatment of fat deposits: lipectomy concerns only the underlying fat, just beneath the resected skin, and the defatting of the remaining flap with a scalpel is a delicate and dangerous procedure that could compromise the vitality of the flap. Although surgical procedures could deal with cutaneous and musculoaponeurotic lesions, the surgical treatment of excess fat was limited to the fatty tissue immediately beneath the distended and damaged skin. The adjoining hypertrophic fat deposits were just sandwiched between the tightened skin and the muscular layer. This fatty inertia was partially responsible for the occasional unsatisfactory results and for any recurrence.

No single surgical procedure could have been proposed for dealing with isolated excess abdominal fat deposits without cutaneous distension.

Liposuction was introduced into the authors' repertoire in 1977, following the work of Illouz. It seems to be the appropriate procedure for the treatment of localized fat excess, and has added a new chapter to the history of plastic surgery of the abdomen.

The possible anatomical applications of this method are many, but it should be considered neither as a self-sufficient technique, nor as an alternative to classic surgery as far as abdominoplasty is concerned. It is rather a means or an instrument to be added to other cutaneous and muscular procedures.

Liposuction makes classic procedures easier since it lessens the fat excess of the flaps, making their mobilization easier. It harmonizes the thickness of the edges to be approximated and diminishes the tension on the sutures, improving the quality of the scars and reducing the dog ears.

Liposuction is carried out first when associated with dermolipectomy. It is an easy procedure that does not lengthen surgery. It is not aggressive on the skin and requires no special postoperative care, unless the volume of aspirated fat is more than one litre.

Although it is easy, liposuction presents a possible accidental complication — that of aponeurotic or peritoneal perforation, with the risk of intraabdominal visceral lesions. Great care should be taken, especially when abdominal scars are present, since they can be very fragile.

Isolated abdominal liposuction (Fig. 8.59)

This is designed for patients with abdominal fat excess located beneath a tonic, undamaged and non-excessive skin, that will spontaneously retract over the new contours.

Before the advent of liposuction, these patients were denied surgery. Today, when the indications are right, they are the ones who will benefit most from abdominoplasty, since their problem can be treated permanently and without scarring.

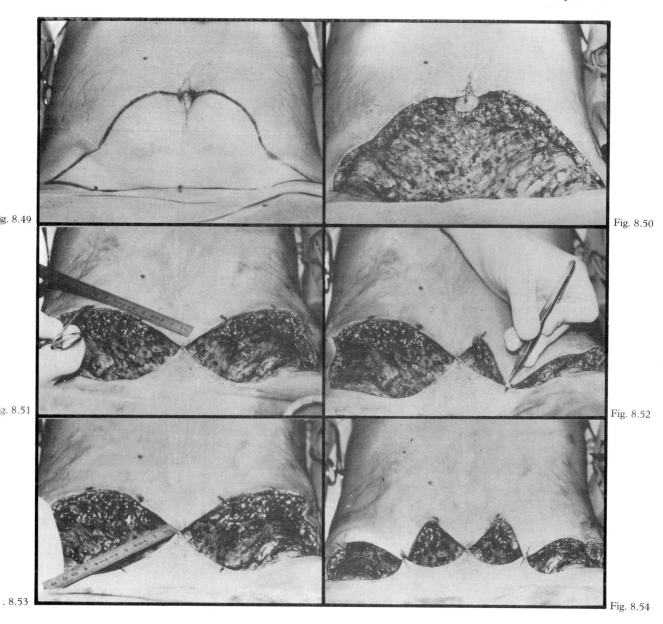

Fig. 8.49

Fig. 8.50

Fig. 8.51

Fig. 8.52

8.53

Fig. 8.54

Fig. 8.49 Symmetrical drawing done in a standing position.

Fig. 8.50 After the excision of the fatty cutaneous excess, an incongruity of the edges is seen.

Fig. 8.51 The 5 cm 'intervals' are marked on the superior edge, on each side of the midline.

Fig. 8.52 The maximum 'cheating' value is evaluated (here, a 10 cm interval). A mark is placed on the lower edge and then measured (6.5 cm for 10 cm in this case: a gain of almost 2 cm for every 5 cm).

Fig. 8.53 Projection of the 'cheating' on the inferior contralateral edge with a rule.

Fig. 8.54 The two symmetrical stay stitches are placed.

Fig. 8.55 Intermediate stitches are placed at the middle of each interval dividing the 'cheating' in an equal manner. A new 5 cm interval is marked.

Fig. 8.56 The transferring of the cheating onto the contralateral edge.

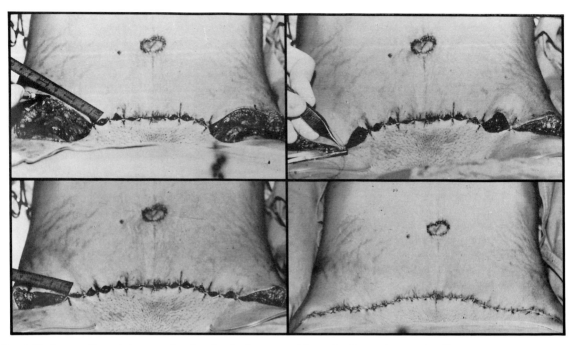

Fig. 8.57 Intermediate stitches are placed and a final interval, 4 cm in this case, is marked.

Fig. 8.58 Front view result. (Figs 8.48 to 8.58 from G. Flageul and E. Sitbon, Ann. Chir. Plast. Esth. 32, 3:223–226, 1987).

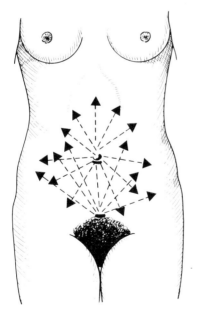
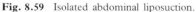
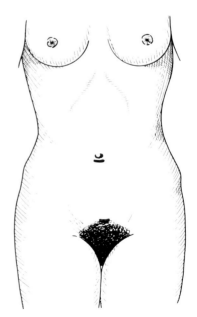

Fig. 8.59 Isolated abdominal liposuction.

Combined dermolipectomy and abdominal liposuction (Figs 8.60–8.66)

When there is localized fat excess all dermolipectomies could benefit from associated liposuction. This can be assessed by an inspection and a pinch test. Liposuction should also be associated with cutaneous reduction plasty in order to adapt the skin covering to the new underlying contours. Dermal lipectomy very often permits the elimination of skin lesions such as stretchmarks and scars.

As far as the umbilicus is concerned, the procedure will depend on the extent and site of the lesions and the amount of excess skin. The many different options available have already been discussed.

Liposuction should be performed at the beginning (primary liposuction) or during the operation. The 'rolling test' permits the control, during the operation, of the thickness of the residual fatty layer and the evenness of the liposuction. The classic abdominoplasty procedures are carried out after this. They are made easier, as has been seen, by the thinning of the superior flap and the elimination of the incongruity of the edges.

Dermolipectomy and liposuction as two separate procedures

This concerns a dermal lipectomy performed in order to correct a residual skin excess a few months after liposuction for which the mechanical qualities of the skin were overestimated. Alternatively, the liposuction could be carried out after the abdominoplasty, in order to complete its action on the fatty layer.

Abdominal dermolipectomy associated with extraabdominal liposuction

A common example of this procedure would be abdominoplasty carried out in association with the liposuction of subtrochanteric fat deposits.

TIGHTENING OF THE MUSCULOAPONEUROTIC LAYER

The treatment of abnormalities of the fatty layer has undergone tremendous change during the last few decades. Treatment of the musculoaponeurotic layer has also progressed. The classic procedures for the treatment of diastasis recti (plication of the rectus at the midline by a series

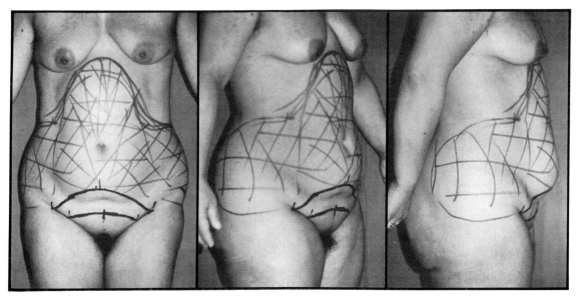

Figs 8.60, 8.61 and 8.62 Low transverse dermolipectomy with liposuction and without an umbilical procedure marking of the resection and liposuction areas.

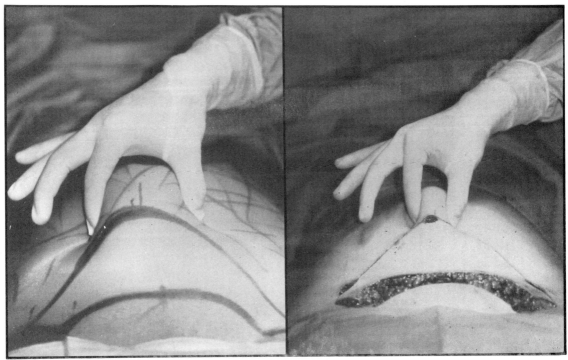

Figs 8.63 and 8.64   Evaluation of the amount of fatty tissue before and after liposuction. The liposuction was performed before the cutaneous resection.

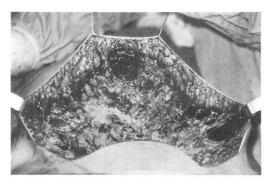

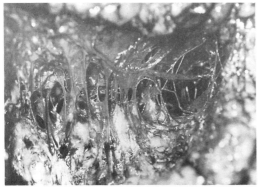

Figs 8.65 and 8.66   Typical aspect of the 'fatty tunnels'.

of buried sutures (Welti–Quénu procedure)) will be described briefly in Chapter 10 (Figs 8.67, 8.68).

There is a recent therapeutic approach based on the observation of muscular and aponeurotic distensions and loosenings that are detrimental to the figure and to the abdominal wall, outwith classic lesions such as eventration, hernia and diastasis. The treatment of such distensions stems from the same concern for the superficial musculoaponeurotic structures in the ageing of the face and in lifting. Two therapeutic orientations seem to be of interest:

1. Jackson, in 1978, described a biaxial plication which he called a 'waistline stitch'. It seemed to him that there is a musculoaponeurotic loosening following a vertical line extending from the xiphoid to the pubis, associated with the diastasis recti. Jackson proposed to associate the classic vertical plication of the rectus with a horizontal transverse plication involving the external and internal oblique and the

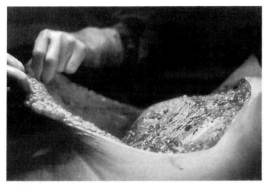

Fig. 8.67 Important diastasis recti. J. S. Elbaz and G. Flageul.

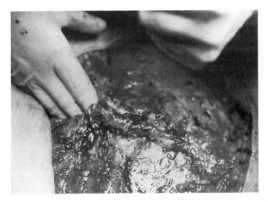

Fig. 8.68 Treatment of the diastasis recti with a series of X-shaped buried sutures.

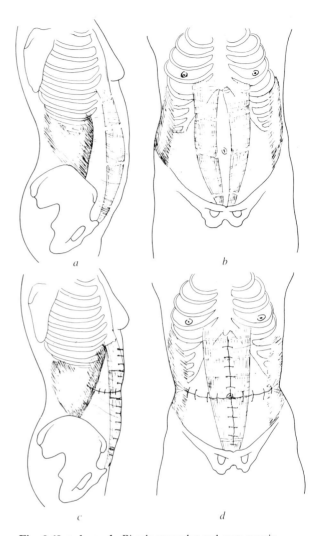

a   *b*

c   *d*

Fig. 8.69 a, b, c, d Bi-axle muscular and aponeurotic plication according to Jackson (1978).

transversus abdominis muscles, crossing at the umbilicus (Fig. 8.69).

2. In the same year, and following the same principle, Psillakis proposed a plication of the external oblique to the external margin of the rectus sheath.

DIFFERENT PROCEDURES FOR THE UMBILICUS

Recent progress in abdominal plastic surgery has also been marked by a number of new surgical techniques for the umbilicus, such as disinsertion or resection, on reconstructions and improvements of existing procedures such as umbilical transposition or plasty.

As far as abdominoplasty is concerned, the umbilicus is anatomically and technically in the centre of the subject, as are the nipple and areola in mammoplasty. However, the nipple and areola are major and complex anatomical structures; the umbilicus is simply a scar. This unique cicatricial nature explains the diversity of the methods that can be used for the umbilicus without changing its shape. A thorough knowledge of these methods is essential, and this section will consider umbilical transposition, disinsertion resection-reconstruction, and umbilicoplasty.

Umbilical transposition

This is really a pseudotransposition since the umbilicus does not change place. The stump can be moved up or down by 1–2 cm.

There are various different methods for umbilical transposition. Flesh, Thebesius and Wheishmer (1931) were the first to approach this concept. They transposed a cutaneous equilateral triangle centred on the umbilicus in a low transverse abdominoplasty, but it is to Mornard (1938) and Vernon (1957) that we owe the first descriptions of the transposition of an isolated umbilical ring. This is one of the most used procedures in abdominoplasty, consisting of a horizontal cutaneous incision at the projection of the umbilicus, allowing its exteriorization.

Other incisions have been proposed for the exteriorization of the umbilical ring: vertical, fusiform and figure-of-eight. These procedures will not be discussed here; rather it will be shown what can be done to improve the periumbilical scar. Two propositions seem to be of interest here.

1. In 1978, Avelar proposed a method of replacing the circular periumbilical scar by a star-shaped scar hidden in the umbilicus itself (Fig. 8.70a,b,c). The umbilicus is isolated and dissected following a three-branched star plan rather than a circular one. After locating the area of umbilical projection on the lowered upper abdominal flap, a circle 2 cm in diameter is drawn: it is then divided with a scalpel into three equilateral triangular flaps that open like a star. Next, three central umbilical flaps are made that will interpose naturally between the three abdominal flaps

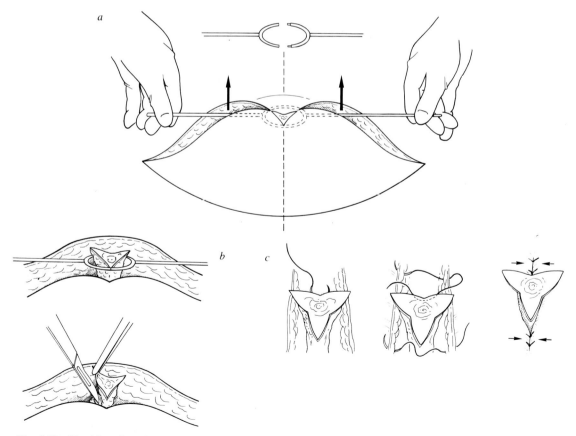

Fig. 8.70 The 'three-branch star drawing' in umbilical transposition. (J. M. Avelar).

just created, and all are sutured together. The result is a natural-looking umbilicus, with a star-shaped scar hidden inside it.

2. Juri (1979) proposed a similar but easier method: an incision is made on the upper abdominal flap following the right and left sides of an equilateral triangle with its base uppermost. Its vertex corresponds to the point of exteriorization. The incision of the umbilicus follows its median upper radius. The final scar is only partially periumbilical (about 270°); the remaining 90° is replaced by two scars hidden within the umbilicus.

It is important to defat the abdominal flap around the incision that was made for exteriorizing the umbilicus. This is more important above the opening than below, as it will then permit the new umbilicus to be placed at the bottom of a depression.

Umbilical disinsertion

Umbilical disinsertion avoids the transposition that forces the supraumbilical point to become suprapubic. It does not involve any extra mid-abdominal scarring. Umbilical disinsertion with low transverse abdominoplasty has already been described.

Umbilical resection–reconstruction

This is also known as neoumbilicoplasty, and is indicated when the umbilicus is missing (for example in patients who have undergone laparotomy), or when resection rather than transposition of the umbilicus is preferred. It is a functional indication in the obese patient with an umbilical hernia or a diastasis recti. The resected umbilicus should then be reconstructed. Several procedures have been described for this:
In 1978, Sabatier proposed an easy method consisting of creating two opposing U-shaped flaps at the chosen site for the new umbilicus. The deep side of these two flaps should be carefully defatted at the portion of the dermis that will constitute the bottom. This amounts to a conical excision of the fatty tissue just beneath the skin of the future umbilical site. The flaps are then sutured together and to the aponeurosis. The

bare skin, applied directly to the aponeurosis of the linea alba, adheres to it and forms a cicatricial depression, anatomically similar to a natural umbilicus.

Following the same principle and procedures, other techniques have been described using three or four flaps (V-shaped quadruple plasty with a central vertex; Fig. 8.71).

Fournier proposed an even easier technique. This consists of a transverse arc-shaped incision, perfectly centred on the midline and measuring 3 cm. It should be defatted along the edges, especially the upper one, to create a median supraumbilical depression. Both sides of the incision are then sutured to the aponeurotic surface below. The shape of the new umbilicus is maintained for a few days with the application of a Biogaze bolus.

Umbilicoplasty

It is unusual to change the morphology of the umbilicus, but it could be useful for a large and protruding umbilicus. Hodgkinson, in 1983, proposed a technique inspired by the neo-umbilicoplasty technique, using two flaps. The umbilicus is pulled out with a surgical hook, and two flaps, an inferior and a superior, are dissected from the umbilical skin. The superior flap should be twice as long as the inferior one. The protruding umbilical scar is then resected and any parietal defects are corrected. The superior flap is partially plicated and its distal side sutured to the aponeurotic surface. The inferior flap fits naturally in place and is sutured to the superior flap and to the aponeurotic surface.

COMBINATION OF OTHER SURGERY WITH ABDOMINOPLASTY

Different possibilities can be considered, depending on the type of surgery, particularly on whether or not the peritoneum is opened.

Combination with another plastic surgical procedure

Although plastic surgery of the abdomen is not a minor operation, it could logically be associated

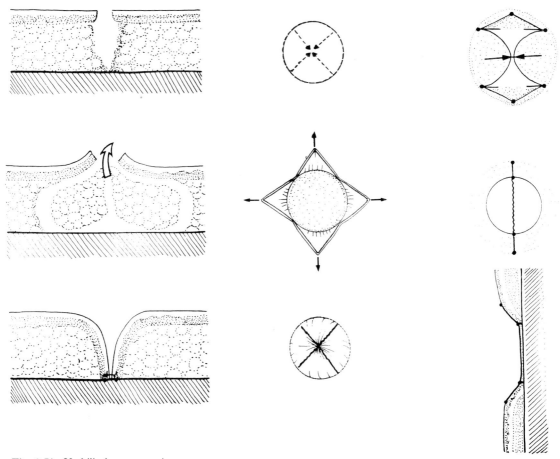

Fig. 8.71 Umbilical reconstruction.

with another plastic surgical procedure. Often this will be a mammoplasty. Cardoso de Castro in 1978 reported a series of 30 abdominoplasties and reduction mammoplasties performed at the same operation, with a postoperative progress comparable to simple abdominoplasty.

Other combinations of surgery are possible but care should be taken not to lengthen the operative time too much. The medicolegal aspects of combining surgical procedures should also be considered.

Combination with treatment of eventration

This is a logical combination, since all muscular and aponeurotic lesions and fatty-cutaneous disorders can be treated at the same time. However, in the case of major eventration necessitating the opening of the peritoneum or the placement of a prosthesis, especially in an obese patient, the detachment should be limited and small.

Combination with visceral abdominal surgery

This is a delicate situation. The treatment of an intraabdominal visceral lesion, should be separate from abdominoplasty for security reasons: it is a matter of 'proportionality'. Several publications and daily practice have somehow modified this rule. Each case, then, should be considered separately according to different parameters. If the patient is in good health, and if the surgeries are performed by two different surgical teams, the combination of parietal surgery with an intraabdominal procedure is a possibility.

Surgeons should remain very cautious. In 1986, Voss published a series of 76 combinations of abdominoplasty with gynaecological surgery; He reported pulmonary embolism in 6.6% of the cases. This is much higher than after an isolated abdominoplasty or an isolated hysterectomy. He isolates a high-risk group — women over 50 and weighing over 70 kg.

9. Liposuction

The purpose of liposuction is to remove the fatty tissue and the fatty cells, with minimal scarring and no recurrence. It preserves the blood vessels and avoids the creation of a single cavity or the formation of cutaneous 'waves'. In 1986, 100 000 liposuctions were performed in the United States (ASPS statistics) almost as many as face-lifts. The great contribution that liposuction has made to cosmetic surgery should be acknowledged.

HISTORY

Schrudde originally had the idea of removing subcutaneous fat with a sharp uterine curette; however, the abrasion was too superficial, the results were too uncertain and deep necrosis was always a possibility.

In 1977, Fischer described the Italian method for dealing with 'riding breeches': from a 3 cm incision directly over the fatty mass, a complete detachment is performed with long scissors. The fatty mass is then ground with an electric cutter and aspirated. The author himself reported the high incidence of haematomas, of infection, and especially of seromas necessitating drainage for several weeks and sometimes several months. Also the skin would slide over the deep layer because of the impossibility of the two surfaces of the cavity joining. This caused Vilain to comment that the operation 'transformed riding breeches into golf trousers'.

Kiesselring, in 1978, described his technique using a cannula of his own devising that had a sharp pointed end. Although this is a tunnelling technique, visual examination of the work carried out by the catheter frequently demonstrates the creation of a single cavity and vascular damage.

Illouz, also in 1978, gave his first paper on his new surgical technique for localized lipodistrophy. There were four main principles:

1. To use an atraumatic cannula with one hole, or several holes located at least 1.5 cm from the blunt tip of the instrument.
2. To proceed by tunnelling. This avoids the creation of a single cavity. The vessels and the perforating nerves move away from the cannula and are thus preserved.
3. To preserve the superficial fatty tissue (Avelar's upper layer) above the superficial fascia. It has been seen that this fatty tissue is normal, that it contains the main lymphatic vessels and allows the patient to gain or lose weight harmoniously. Only the localized fatty tissue, that responsible for the deformation of the figure, should be treated.
4. To assess the plasticity of the skin (elasticity and retraction power) depending on the abundance of fat to be aspirated. All skin excess results in an unsightliness at least equal to the initial problem.

The principle behind this technique is to create several tunnels in the fatty mass, which when compressed, and assisted by lymphatic drainage, will heal by fibrosis, significantly reducing the thickness of the fatty mass.

The opposite of liposuction, the reinjection of aspirated fat (filling), is very controversial although it is practised in Brazil and in the United States.

In 1984, the first observations of Illouz on this subject were met with a good deal of scepticism. Although it is certain that fatty cells cannot multiply or even survive independently, it seems that the culture and reinjection of a prefatty cell that can survive and reproduce in vitro (Berland, Lafontan and Costagliola) could lead to some very fruitful research.

THEORETICAL BASIS

Chemical and physical studies have shown no difference between the subcutaneous fatty tissue situated above the superficial fascia, and the fat of fat deposits. However, given the current state of knowledge of cellular chemistry, these results seem to be a little premature.

Why is it that when a woman gains weight, the fat accumulates at certain preferential sites, and when she loses weight, it disappears last from these same sites? This is the big mystery about fatty cells.

Fatty cells

These are programmed to store energy in the form of triglycerides that can be used when needed. They derive from the prefatty cells of mesodermal origin that proliferate from birth and then start to differentiate. They are then transformed into fatty cells and stop dividing. Under the electron microscope, the fatty cells appear free from one another; they present as either a large lipidic inclusion or several smaller ones, occupying most of the cell and pushing the nucleus against the cellular membrane. In humans, the fatty cells use the circulating triglyceride of hepatic or intestinal origin (chylomicrons). These circulating triglycerides are hydrolysed by the action of lipase into fatty acids, and then resynthesized by the fatty cells into personal triglycerides.

It is a problem to know whether the removal of these fat deposits is dangerous or not for the organism, as they 'pump out' the circulating triglycerides, and because of the resulting high risk of hyperlipoproteinaemia.

The slight importance of the genetic code in determining the number of subcutaneous fat cells allows us to better understand lipoatrophy or thinness. Obesity, which is a symptom and not a disease, is due to an increase in size of the fatty cells (hypertrophic obesity) and severe obesity is due to the increase in the number of fatty cells (hyperplastic obesity).

Bjornstorp's fatty cell theory

Based on animal experimentation, the principle behind this is that we are born with a certain number of fatty cells that are able to store the circulating fat. These cells multiply and proliferate until puberty, and then stop, their number remaining the same (they can multiply exceptionally in the case of morbid obesity). This explains the importance of the age of reference and the weight of an individual, immediately after puberty; and the mechanism of all slimming treatments: the cells lose some of their intracellular triglycerides; they actually become thinner. However, when the diet is over, they are ready to fatten up again, or even more so, having undergone a (for them) unusual diet.

The problem is knowing whether this theory, obtained from experimentation on adult rats, is valid for humans. It can be said that 80% of all obesities are hypertrophic (same cell numbers but high storage capacity). In this case, the destruction of fatty cells cannot be followed by recurrence since the quantity of cells has diminished. This is a good indication for liposuction. However, in the remaining 20% the obesity is hyperplastic; this means that the fatty cells could multiply and the destruction of some of them would not help at all.

Alpha and beta receptors

The recent work of Harner, Berlan and Lafontan has shown that the fatty cell is sensitive to two kinds of receptors: β_1 that leads to lipolysis, and α_2 that blocks lipolysis. These receptors are sensitive to the same neuroreceptors, adrenalin and noradrenalin — two catecholamines with a double alpha and beta potentiality.

Lipolytic beta-adrenergic receptors

These have been known for 20 years. The metabolism of triglyceride hydrolysis is as follows: the binding of the hormone to a beta receptor leads to the activation of a membrane enzyme, adenyl-cyclase. This enzyme catalyses the transformation of ATP into AMPC (messenger), which activates the protein kinase. This in turn activates a hormone-sensitive lipase, hydrolysing the triglycerides into fatty acids and glycerol.

It seems that there is no major malfunctioning of this system in the fatty tissue of obese people, but we know that the lipolytic action of adrenalin and noradrenalin is less than that of isoprenalin. The systematic exploration of the adrenergic receptors of the different fat deposits has shown that the subcutaneous fatty cells of the outer side of the thigh (riding breeches) are resistant to the lipolytic action of adrenalin. The functional variations of the different localizations of fat deposits could be explained by the variable alpha-antilipolytic adrenergic effect. The question is whether these receptors are involved in obesity, and more precisely, in resistance to losing weight.

The characteristics of α_2 receptors

These are very active in localized fat deposits, especially 'riding breeches'. This could explain why a woman can lose weight from all over her body apart from fat deposits such as 'riding breeches', where α_2 blocks lipolysis considerably. The destruction of fatty cells and α_2 receptors in these areas eliminates the lipolysis-blocking agents, allowing the patient to lose weight if dieting. There is no recurrence and vasodilation and a rise in the temperature of the lower limb have frequently been noted.

LIPOSUCTION EQUIPMENT

This consists of the following:
A suction pump. This has a high-power engine with an output of 120 l/min of air. It can produce a negative pressure of 1 kg/cm² . It is attached on

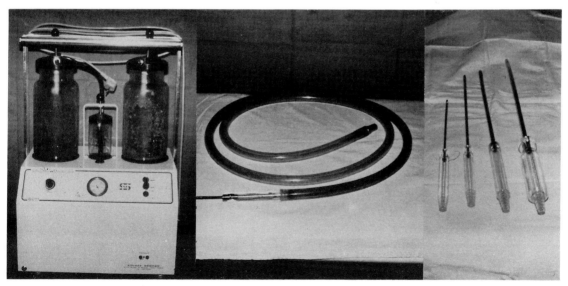

Fig. 9.1   Fig. 9.2   Fig. 9.3

Fig. 9.1 The suction pump with its bottles.

Fig. 9.2 The hose.

Fig. 9.3 The cannulas with their transparent handle, and a diameter going from 8–10 mm to 2 mm.

one side to one or two sterile bottles and on the other side to a heavy-duty transparent hose of 1.5–2 cm diameter, to which a series of cannulas can be fitted (Figs 9.1, 9.2).

The cannulas (Fig. 9.3). Their handles are either metallic or made out of transparent material. They have a mark for the thumb that corresponds to the holes on the shaft: These should always be 'looking' towards the deep layer. This thumb mark is very important and all cannulas have one. *The shafts.* These are 25–50 cm long and have a diameter of 4–10 mm. The tip is always blunt and round. The hole is at least 1.5 cm from the tip in order to preserve the thickness of the sub-cutaneous panniculus (between 1 and 1.5 cm of subcutaneous fatty tissue should be left, in order to avoid the formation of 'waves'). Some cannulas have several orifices.

DRY METHOD AND WET METHOD

The fatty tissue can be treated without previous injection: this is the dry method.

The wet method of Illouz uses 3 cm deep injections, each 5 cm apart. The injected solution consists of 20 cm^3 distilled water, 100 UI hyaluronidase and 0.5 mg adrenalin per 500 cm^3 physiological water. These injections are supposed to break up the cellular membrane. The authors disagree, but this wet method has at least three advantages:

1. It produces a hydrodissection after 15–25 minutes.
2. It makes liposuction easier.
3. The adrenalin helps the aspiration of a pure yellow fatty tissue. When this becomes bloody, the operator should change to another tunnel. This is very important.

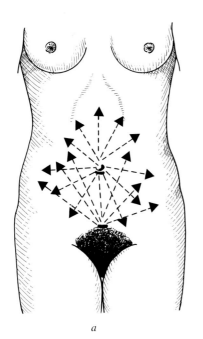 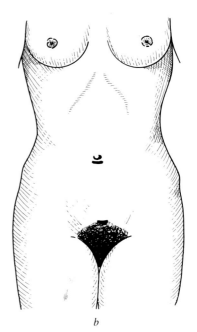

a   *b*

Fig. 9.4 a and b The different approaches. The drawing shows the star-shaped ways where the cannulas should pass.

The best results of liposuction are obtained in the sub-umbilical region. Liposuction should be performed with great care in the epigastric and supra-umbilical region, considering the low retraction ability of the skin at this level. The fatty tissue is very different from that of the sub-umbilical area.

The liposuction allows the diminution of fat deposits from the lateral side of the flanks without increasing the scar length.

With adequate post-operative care a volume going from 500–2500 mls could be aspirated.

THE DIFFERENT APPROACHES (Fig. 9.4)

For the abdomen these are umbilical; in the pubic triangle, where it will be hidden; this can be completed by two small incisions at the anterior–superior iliac spines (Figs 9.5–9.7).

ANAESTHESIA

This depends on the amount of fatty tissue to be aspirated. Up to 500 g, local anaesthesia plus adrenalin or neuroleptanalgesia can be used, always with an anaesthetist present and in a clinic or a hospital. From 500–1500 g, liposuction should be performed under general or epidural anaesthesia. In either case fluid losses should be compensated for with macromolecules, usually at least 1 g for each 1 g aspirated.

From 1500–3000 g blood should be available since the problem could be similar to the 'crush syndrome' described by Bywaters. In this case, the vital prognosis could be in jeopardy. Illouz's recommended treatment for fluid replacement is as follows: before surgery, 1 litre of normal saline; during surgery, and according to the aspirated volume, 50% normal saline, 25% macromolecules and 25% blood.

Fig. 9.5 a and b The clinical evaluation is very important. Ask the patient to retract her abdomen. This gives an exact idea of the result of an isolated liposuction.

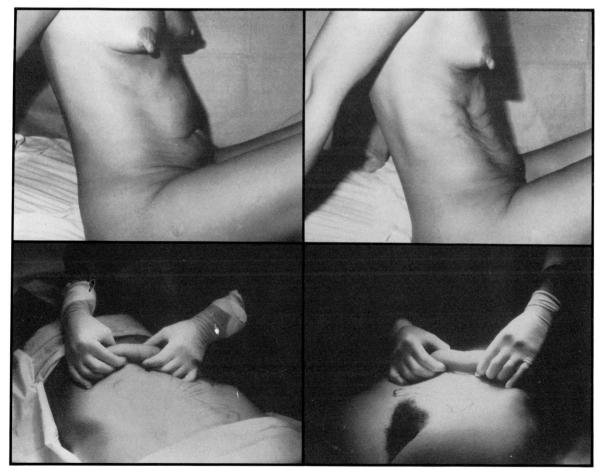

Fig. 9.6 Pinching test.

Fig. 9.7 Rolling test.

THE TECHNIQUE

The movement should be perfectly regular, beginning with the large cannulas (8 mm, for example) and finishing with the small ones (4 mm). A right-handed surgeon should hold the cannula with his right hand and use an in-and-out movement, while using his left hand to hold the fatty panniculus in front of the tip of the cannula and feeling the decrease in thickness of the fatty mass. The pinch test should give 2 cm between the thumb and the index, equal to 1 cm subcutaneously.

The roll test allows the evenness of the work to be felt. Also if the left hand presses the cannula against the deep layer, its position in relation to the skin can be estimated. In any case, the thumb mark on the shaft indicates that the holes are facing the deep layer.

The cannula will work directly on the fat deposits (previously marked on the conscious patient), concentrating on the highest points and moving away from them with decreasing intensity; it will also follow the tunnels corresponding to the different arrows marked on the abdominal wall, starting at the incision and covering the whole abdominal area. These tunnels are not only distributed at the surface but also at different levels of the deep layer (one should always have in mind the image of a Swiss cheese).

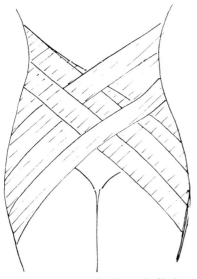

Fig. 9.8 Dressing made by P. Regnault: X shaped elastoplast dressing that relieves suturing tension.

The operator should change from one tunnel to another as soon as there is blood on the shaft or in the tube. Tunnels can intersect, starting from different incisions such as the umbilical or pubic ones.

Great care should be taken not to aspirate the supraumbilical fatty tissue, since this is different in texture and density from the subumbilical fat.

The liquid collected into the two bottles (each corresponding to one of the two sides) has three layers, easily seen after a 15-minute sedimentation. From top to bottom these are pure triglycerides; yellow fatty tissue, made out of fatty cells, 30% of which are still alive; aspirated blood. This last should be as little as possible.

In this manner liposuction permits a real 'defatting' of the abdominal wall, either performed separately (pure abdominal liposuction) or performed first during an abdominoplasty, when it facilitates the surgical procedure, reduces the detachment area and preserves the perforating vascular and nervous pedicle. It also allows the removal of fatty deposits on the sides, and the slimming of the waist, which has practically obviated three-quarter anterior lipectomies. It allows the correction of 'dog ears' without additional cutaneous resection, and it makes the residual scar very much shorter.

Finally, it is possible to perform liposuction on the buttocks, the neck and the inner side of the thighs and for 'riding breeches'.

DRESSING AND POSTOPERATIVE CARE

Dressing is done on the operating table with a 'lipo-panty', of which different brands and sizes are available. They should go from under the rib cage to just above the knees (Figs 9.8, 9.9), and should be worn night and day for a month. Additional physiotherapy, such as pressotherapy and lymphatic drainage, should be performed by a physiotherapist starting on the tenth day, three times weekly for a month.

After the operation and for the first 48 hours, the patient may feel dizzy and should remain under medical observation by the anaesthetist. Asthenia is common during the first month following liposuction.

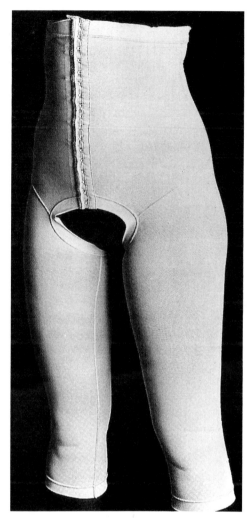

Fig. 9.9 Lipo-Panty, (Medical Z).

Ecchymosis is present for 2–3 weeks. Some patients complain of pain of variable intensity.

The treated area is oedematous for 6 weeks to 2 months. This conceals the result, and the patient should be warned. It is only at the end of the second month that the final results and the technical errors (if there are any) can be seen.

Dysesthesia is possible, but usually disappears after 3–6 months.

Technical errors

If there are any technical errors, the result will be unattractive and the patient will notice this even more than the surgeon, since he has only a front and a side view.

Errors can cause dimples, depression grooves, successive irregularities, or 'waves', asymmetrical, volume and contours, suction excess, and insufficient correction. Such results are almost always irreversible, and treatment should be essentially preventive, hence the importance of the preoperative assessment of the skin elasticity. The patient should be asked to retract her abdomen — to 'swallow it' – in order to visualize the postoperative appearance after an isolated liposuction. This is the muscular inspection test. The area should be grasped and pushed in a centripetal fashion. This will show possible future defects.

More technical points:
1. Draw the pattern markings of each fat deposit on the conscious patient in the following areas: supraumbilical, subumbilical, and on the sides if necessary.
2. Mark the tunnels' paths, starting from the incision.
3. Proceed with the liposuction in a regular fashion.
4. Control what is done continuously with the pinch and roll tests.
5. Change tunnels on the surface and in the deep layer.
6. Start with the large cannulas, refining the work by using gradually smaller and smaller cannulas.

Dimples are caused by a subcutaneous and very superficial 'cannula blow'. The 'ski-tip'-shaped cannula protects the superficial fatty tissue from being aspirated. Grooves are caused by very superficial tunnels. Waves are due to a series of grooves resulting from an irregular and badly-oriented movement. The creased appearance of the skin is caused by a poor preoperative assessment of the plasticity of the skin. The curative treatment is very delicate. However for insufficient suction, a small 'touch-up' under local anaesthesia will solve the problem. Skin excess can be corrected with a secondary abdominoplasty.

It is very difficult to fill in a loss of substance. Fatty tissue reinjection, known as 'filling', could improve this defect but not much is known about this procedure and its future.

INDICATIONS FOR LIPOSUCTION AND ABDOMINOPLASTY

The abdominal region is a difficult site for liposuction compared to other, easier, regions such as 'riding breeches', the inner side of the thighs, the hips, the buttocks and the neck. This is a region that does not 'forgive': any error will be visible. The patient sees it daily and will become dissatisfied. This is why, in the authors' opinion, isolated liposuction is indicated for only one type of patient: the young woman with a really positive skin plasticity test, to whom can be shown the result that she could expect from liposuction, by asking her to 'swallow her belly', and who is satisfied with this result.

She should have a good figure and a regular subumbilical fat deposit shaped like half a buoy.

For all other cases of abdominal obesity — being both supra- and subumbilical, with a side extension and with a skin that has lost its plasticity and that will not 'follow' the suppression of a significant volume — liposuction should be combined with abdominoplasty. The operative protocol will be as follows:

1. Primary liposuction.
2. Surgical abdominoplasty with excision of the excess skin.
3. Verification of the deep vascular and nervous pedicle that looks like a 'spider's web'.
4. Complete haemostasis if necessary.
5. Complete the lipectomy of the superior and lateral flap.
6. Correct all thickness disparity and unevenness of the flap with surgical scissors.
7. Tighten the abdominal wall after skin resection and restore to normal tension.
8. Drainage, if the dead space due to undermining is not eliminated with fibrin glue. This will be discussed in Chapter 10.

In conclusion it can be said that an isolated liposuction associated with abdominoplasty in a young woman with a positive muscular inspection test, with regular fat deposits, and with little fat deposit visible when reclining or in a vertical position, but very visible in a sitting position or when leaning forward, can give spectacular results.

10. The standard operation

Two types of operation will be described: low abdominoplasty with umbilical transposition, and cosmetic suction abdominoplasty, or CSA.

LOW TRANSVERSE ABDOMINOPLASTY WITH UMBILICAL TRANSPOSITION

Like any other surgical procedure, abdominoplasty should follow strict rules. Two very important factors should be stressed.

The somatic factor. This is particularly important in the case of an obese patient, since obesity should be considered as a debilitating factor exposing the patient to postoperative complications, particularly with primary liposuction.

The psychological factor. This applies mostly in the case of a request for cosmetic surgery. Whatever the motivation, the final result should be morphologically superior to the presenting condition.

Preoperative assessment

Problems vary with the type of patient; for instance, treating a flaccid and distended abdomen in a young woman requires a complete preoperative clinical and biological assessment, but above all, a long discussion with the patient in order to discern her motives for surgery. The principles of the operation must be carefully explained and the technique outlined in a way the patient can easily understand. It is essential to emphasize that the resulting scars will remain unattractive and obvious for at least a year; that it will take a long time before they become acceptable and that they will *never* fully disappear.

The operation should never be minimized; the patient should be told that there are no small operations and that any surgical intervention involves a risk.

The scar lines should be drawn with a marking pencil, so that the patient can see what is involved.

The surgeon should criticize 'hyperaesthetic' operations, excessively discreet lesions, and patients who have an obvious disproportion between physical deformities and psychological reactions, who believe a miracle can be performed with plastic surgery. The patient must give fully informed consent before any operation takes place. It is possible that such informed consent has no legal value whatsoever, but it does constitute a warning for those patients who may expect too much.

The problem of dermolipectomy, especially combined with primary liposuction, is different. This is a major operation, and the risks must be realized and evaluated by preliminary consultation with the anaesthetist who will handle the patient. Needless to say, the surgeon should refuse to operate on the high-risk patient.

History-taking

This is to ascertain:

1. Age, occupation, number of pregnancies.
2. Personal history, including onset of obesity and study of its possible causes.
3. Family and past history of obesity, diabetes or arterial hypertension.
4. Hygienic and dietary habits, especially eating habits and muscular activity.

5. Diets and treatment already followed. People who want to lose weight at all costs have many tricks and will resort to anything, including thyroid extracts, often hidden within homeopathic products, diuretics which cause a loss of potassium, anorectics and antidepressants.

6. Psychological profile: the patient's motivation and preconceived ideas about the operation.

7. The physical price to be paid in terms of scarring. It must be stressed that a known deformity will be replaced by an unknown deformity, albeit temporarily.

Clinical examination

Note must be made of the following:

1. Type of obesity: localized, generalized, gynoid or android.

2. Measurements of the patient's maximum weight, minimum weight, present weight and its duration; also the Livi index, based on the weight/height ratio of the subject.

3. Cardiopulmonary status, not only arterial pressures and cardiac examination but also respiratory problems often encountered among obese patients.

4. Grading (with the patient in a prone position) of the abdominal musculature. This gives an opportunity to look for diastasis, hernia and eventration.

5. Status of the veins in the legs, especially a history of previous phlebitis.

6. Endocrine problems.

Additional examinations

These include:

1. Glucogenic assessment: provoked glycaemia and hyperglycaemia. The frequency of such problems in obese patients is well known.

2. Lipids: cholesterol, total lipids and triglycerides.

3. Cardiorespiratory assessment: electrocardiogram, chest X-ray, and in case of severe obesity, especially with a large eventration, a respiratory function test.

4. In addition to the other common tests (blood grouping, blood typing, urea) a systematic picture of the lumbosacral area must be obtained in order to detect a possible hyperlordosis, which could be the cause of the anterior projection of the abdominal wall. In such a case, as has been seen, the operation will never result in a flat abdomen.

5. Whatever the problem (obesity, stretchmarks, scarred or wrinkled abdomen) an assessment of the abdominal wall should be made, to discover the state of the skin (muscular inspection test), the state of the fatty cutaneous tissue (even thickness or atrophy), the quality of the muscles and the shape of the abdomen (wide or large).

All these parameters will be studied in order to choose the most appropriate technique. The results are recorded on a diagram, which grades the lesions according to the classification suggested in Chapter 4.

Finally, the authors stress the importance of preoperative photographs, which constitute a true medicolegal document.

- Face, profile and three-quarters of the full height of the subject with the forearms away from the hips.
- Close-up of the face, profile and three-quarters centred on the abdomen, framing the breasts and the upper third of the thighs.
- Face, profile and three-quarters, with the patient leaning forward at 45° in order to see and record the degree of ptosis and sagging of the skin.
- Face, profile and three-quarters, with the patient in a sitting position.

PREPARATION OF THE PATIENT

Preparation of the skin

Preparation of the skin is a matter of scientific philosophy. There is frequently a microclimate in the folds of the skin, especially in the inferior fold of a pendulous abdomen, with pigmented lesions, maceration and proliferation of local bacteria. It would be foolhardy to think that such disorders must be corrected at all costs before surgery, since the operation itself will enable a normal oxygenation of the scars, and the lesions will heal within a month.

However, the patient must be bathed before surgery and the skin must be prepared 1 hour before the operation. The authors do not resort to the use of antiseptic solutions, and do not apply postoperative dressings, as they tend to cause heat and humidity which will encourage local bacteria to multiply, rather than reducing them.

Intestinal preparation

Intestinal preparation is useful only in the case of a combined large eventration. It is enough to maintain the patient on a plain, non-residual diet for 2 weeks before the operation. This is better than enemas (which are irritating), antibiotics or the so-called intestinal sulfonamides.

Drawing the incisions and locating fat deposits

The incisions are drawn with a marker on the eve of the operation, with the patient in a standing position; she may be asked to correct any postural defects (shoulders or pelvis; see Fig. 10.1).

A test 'fitting' will follow: the surgeon will hold any excess skin with both hands, looking for the proper direction in which to pull the upper flap (directly to the bottom, downwards and inwards, or downwards and outwards), marking the iliac spines, the xiphopubic line, and cross-ruling the abdomen so as to connect the superior points with the inferior points. Finally the xiphoumbilical distance and the pubic triangle–xiphoid distance are measured. Any increase in the latter will give the measure of excess skin, and hence the quantity of skin to be resected.

THE OPERATION

The three main objectives here are asepsis, rapid execution without undue haste, and meticulous haemostasis.

Position of the patient

The jackknife position is no longer used, since it is unsuitable for liposuction; the patient is placed in the dorsal decubitus position.

Preparation of the operative field

The authors always prepare the entire surface with iodized alcohol, from the breasts to the upper third of the thighs, as well as the sides and the rubber sheet on which the patient has been placed. Sewn drapes, jersey sheets or steridrapes are not used.

Primary liposuction

This will be performed supra- or subumbilically, depending on the case. The technique has been described in Chapter 9.

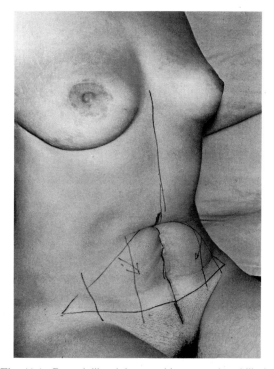

Fig. 10.1 Buttock-like abdomen with a normal umbilical PPT distance of 13 cms; a difficult case, as there is very little skin (S2, S1, M1, A0).

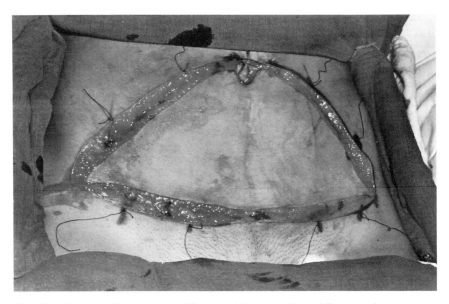

Fig. 10.2 Drawing of the incisions. The scalpel bypasses the umbilicus, the lower incision line, and the upper incision line. Note the cross-markings of the abdomen, done with skinmarking pencil. Sutures are marking the gravity lines of the abdominal cylinder.

The incisions (Fig. 10.1)

The preoperative markings are first traced over with a brush dipped in methylene blue, and the longitudinal periumbilical incision is made, extending slightly above the umbilicus; a number 15 blade is used for this. Using surgical scissors, dissection is carried out from the surface to the deep periumbilical fat; care must be taken to avoid periumbilical necrosis. A larger blade is used to make the lower and upper skin incisions (Fig. 10.2).

The surgeon stands to the right of the patient and the large Museux forceps are placed at the left end of the incision. The two subcutaneous abdominal veins, easily visible, are indentified in the lower pole of the incision and are tied with catgut.

Fatty-cutaneous resection (Fig. 10.3)

The surgeon holds the Museux forceps in his left hand and starts the excision of the fat from the left side of the incision, while the assistant achieves haemostasis of all the vessels with a coagulating forceps. With step-by-step haemostasis accomplished, the dissection continues

across the mid line and proceeds toward the right side of the incision. The small amount of fat remaining on top of the musculoaponeurotic

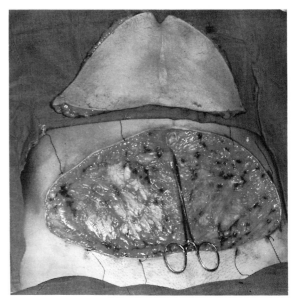

Fig. 10.3 Excision of tissue after rigorous haemostasis. Note the neighbouring superior portion of the flap and its retraction.

plane must be uniform in thickness except in the suprapubic area, where a flute-shaped fatty cushion should be left. When the operation is completed, the subumbilical skin will lie on this, and it will make up for the lack of adipose tissue.

This is a basic resection, based on preoperative measurements and markings. It differs from other techniques, which first incise the inferior line, then dissect and resect as needed. It also differs from the technique of Planas, who proposes the initial incision of the superior line and its dissection and lowering, followed by fatty-cutaneous resection as required.

The advantages of the method described above are its speed of execution and its guaranteed symmetry, because when the skin is pulled, the traction determines the location of the scar; this explains why in other techniques the scars are often poorly placed, even though the surgeon was quite certain of the symmetry of his work during the operation.

However, any error in preoperative planning, such as an overestimated excision, can lead to a catastrophe when suturing begins. This procedure cannot be used by the inexperienced surgeon.

In the case of an adherent scar (appendectomy, subumbilical midline or Pfannenstiel), the dissection of the lower portion of the scar is done carefully to avoid entering the musculo-aponeurotic layer or the peritoneum.

Musculoaponeurotic repairs

In very distended abdomens, the inner aspects of the rectus muscles are plicated in the midline with a series of buried sutures every 1 cm, with size 0 monofilament thread. These sutures include the entire mass of the inner edges of the muscles and their sheaths, without entering the peritoneum. This plication is crucial, as it improves the waist and gives a proper shape to the abdomen (Figs 10.4, 10.5).

Undermining the superior flap (Fig. 10.6)

This detaching process is started with a scalpel. The surgeon then retracts with his left hand, with the aid of a small clamp, and dissects the flaps at their deepest parts, according to the principles

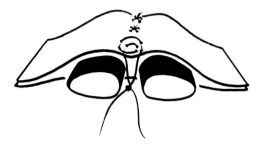

Fig. 10.4 Plication of the rectus at the midline by a series of buried sutures.

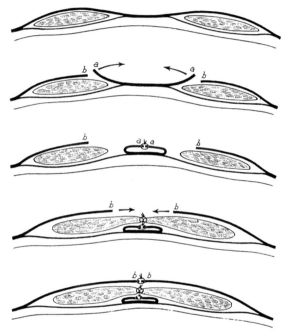

Fig. 10.5 Technique of Edouard Quenu for surgical treatment of a spontaneous eventration by a major diastasis recti (after).

previously mentioned, taking care to preserve the deeper fat. Step-by-step haemostasis is performed, especially of the perforating arteries before their retraction. The detachment is continued almost up to the floating ribs and in the direction of the xiphoid. The surgeon must be sure that the flap is developing well and will approximate to the inferior flap without undue tension.

A Pozzi forceps holds the umbilicus smoothly, and its rings are visible and exteriorized on the inferior flap.

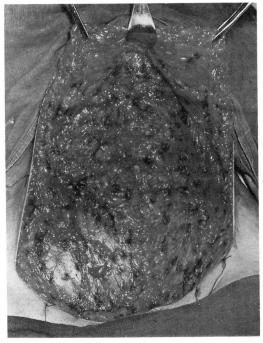

Fig. 10.6 The undermining goes up to the ribs, on the midline, and up to the xyphoid process, which is clearly visible here. It is very important that this undermining be symmetrical.

Sutures (Fig. 10.7)

The authors generally begin with one or two heavy sutures through the entire thickness of the two flaps, on either side of the superior angles of the pubic triangle and the corresponding points of the cross-markings on the upper flap. These sutures are temporary. The subcutaneous stitches approximate the fatty layer edges using buried or inverted catgut mattress sutures, and do not take too large a bite lest they produce adhesions.

The upper flap, which will be anchored to the mons veneris (Glicenstein), is not de-epithelialized. To avoid final adhesions, the fatty-cutaneous levels must be allowed to slide freely over the deepest layer. The permanent location of the sutures is determined not only by bringing the superior flap down but by the combined effects of these factors and by the force exerted on the upper portion of the inferior flap (the raising of the pubic triangle and the external genitalia).

The skin is then approximated from the outside to the inside, allowing the flaps to be perfected when suturing, in order to correct any incongruity of length between the upper and lower flaps. Umbilical exteriorization is the next step.

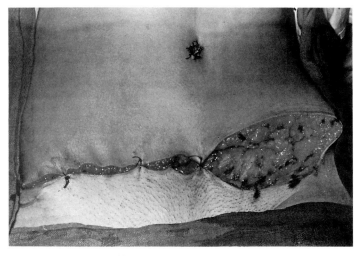

Fig. 10.7 The right half of the incision is approximated by several 'staystitches'. The umbilicus is delivered in a good position, that is, at the level of a tangent drawn at the superior portion of the iliac crest. This is a cleft with a longitudinal excision.

Umbilical exteriorization

The location of the future umbilicus is marked at a point between the xiphopubic line and a transverse tangent at the highest point of the iliac crests. A 1 cm longitudinal incision is made and its lateral edges excised 2–3 mm longitudinally. This area is heavily detatted, as described by Baroudi, so that the umbilicus will not be flush with the skin, but fall into a slight depression with a long vertical axis. Now all that remains is to take the umbilicus, which the assistant holds with the Pozzi forceps, and pull it through the flap, sewing it with U-shaped stitches, the loops being in the umbilical depression.

Drainage

Two Redon drains are placed on either side of the mons pubis and connected to sterile bottles, which will be emptied only once every 24 hours to avoid unnecessary contamination.

Measurement of the new umbilicopubic distance

The new umbilicopubic distance is rarely 13 cm but it may come as close to that as possible (Fig. 10.8)

Dressings

A grease-impregnated dressing is placed on the umbilicus and the suture line and is covered with abdominal pads and a 40 cm wide Velpeau dressing. The patient is taken off the table, being held under the arms and at the knees. Elastoplast bands (8–10 cm wide) are placed crosswise and then in the shape of an X to form a 'girdle' which is perfectly moulded to the body. The authors do not use plaster of Paris, as Pitanguy recommended, nor a sandbag, which would exert pressure on the vessels, is uncomfortable, impedes circulation and does not help haemostasis.

The patient is put carefully back into bed. The foot of the bed is raised, the knees are flexed and held by a soft bolster, and the head is raised on two pillows as soon as possible in order to reduce pressure on the sutures.

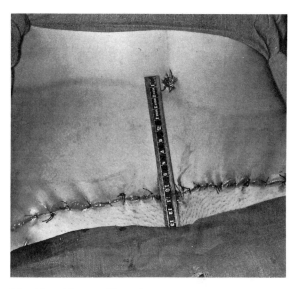

Fig. 10.8 Note: 1. The puboumbilical distance, which here is 10.5 cms, is quite adequate, considering the absence of skin relaxation. 2. The incongruity of the two edges is corrected by a U-suture which is narrow at the bottom and wide at the top. This corrugated look disappears as soon as the structures are removed.

The excised portion of abdominal skin and fat is shown to the patient as early as the following day, and this has an important psychological effect.

Immediate postoperative sequelae

No antibiotics or anticoagulants are prescribed, thus avoiding the possibility of a massive haematoma. On the second and third days haemoglobin, haematocrit and the amount of drainage from the Redon drains (changed only once every 24 hours) must be checked; finally a clinical check should be made when the dressing is changed 48 hours postoperatively.

The most important factor is early ambulation — on the evening of the operation or the next morning, with the assistance of a nurse, especially in the case of controlled hypotension. The drains are removed as soon as they cease to function — draining only a clear fluid or on the 6th or 7th postoperative day at the latest — which is generally the day the patient is discharged. The sutures will be removed on the 15th day at the latest.

Table 10.1 ASA (aesthetic suction abdominoplasty) (J. S. Elbaz, 1974)

This is an operation for small and average size lesions of the abdomen, excess fatty deposits.

Combining:
First suction:
subumbilical
sometimes supraumbilical, being very careful as the fat at this level is of a different texture.

Surgery: after a first intra-follicular pubic incision/excision, the dissection of the subumbilical area is possible and possibly the disinsertion of the umbilicus. Using a fibrin glue simplifies the post-operative state and eliminates detachment.

A scar virtually masked by pubic hair, the ideal being the 'horseshoe' scar.

The authors have always advised the wearing of a small elastic girdle for 1 month postoperatively. Abdominal exercises cannot be done for at least 1 month after surgery.

COSMETIC SUCTION ABDOMINOPLASTY (CSA)

This can be used for the correction of moderate fatty-cutaneous lesions. It is a localized low abdominoplasty utilizing

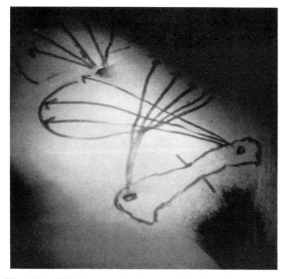

Fig. 10.9 Working area (patient partially shaved).

- Primary liposuction, either supraumbilical from an umbilical incision, or subumbilical from two little intrafollicular pubic incisions;
- A horseshoe incision;
- A double excision, the first being intrapubic, leaving an equilateral pubic triangle each side of which measures 7 cm, and the second in the subumbilical skin;
- With or without umbilical disinsertion allowing to slide 2–3 cm downwards (Fig. 10.9) the supraumbilical and subumbilical fatty-cutaneous plane;
- A fibrin glue, in order to eliminate detachment.

FIBRIN GLUE

Fibrin glue consists of fibrinogen, with factor XIII and aprotinin, and thrombin activated by calcium chloride ions. When combined by spraying, these two constituents will form a natural glue, fibrin, that completes coagulation. It is actually a 're-inforced clot of long lifespan', with variable resorption time. This resorption is due to plasmin and becomes longer (12–15 days, depending on the tissues) under the influence of aprotinin, an antienzyme that inhibits fibrinolysis. Thrombin can be used in concentrations of 500 IU/ml (hardening is almost instantaneous, after 30 s), or 4 IU/ml; here the hardening occurs after approximately 3 minutes, giving enough time to complete the staystitches and the redraping of the skin.

The authors use the 4 IU solution, consisting of human fibrinogen and bovine thrombin. They are guaranteed against any viral contamination, including HIV but not hepatitis B. The product has been available since 1972 and has been used in 1.5 million surgical procedures, not counting plastic and reconstructive surgery. The USFDA has not yet allowed its use in plastic surgery, although it does allow it for cardiovascular surgery.

How to use fibrin glue

The use of fibrin glue requires a fibrinotherm and a double syringe with a common needle (Duploject). The fibrinotherm brings the different constituents to a temperature of 37°C while agitating them electromagnetically.

Spraying is carried out by hooking this double syringe via a three-way valve to a hose equipped with an antiseptic filter and connected to a bottle containing pressurized gas.

The authors use 0.5 cm³ fibrin glue for a 10 × 10 cm quadrilateral; 1, 2, or 3 cm³ are needed per abdominoplasty, depending on the dissected area to be glued. The high price of the product is a real drawback, and many people do not like to use human fibrinogen, although it is highly purified.

A thorough knowledge of the techniques of glueing and draping should be acquired. Spraying should be carried out at a distance of 10 cm from the treated area. For redraping, the skin should be held firmly during the whole glueing and hardening process.

Using fibrin glue has a number of advantages:
1. It eliminates all detachment within 3 minutes.
2. It reinforces haemostasis but cannot restore circulation, and this should be done very carefully. The glue does not stop the bleeding of a perforating artery. Partial haematomas can form on the surface because of poor glueing techniques.
3. By eliminating any deadspace, it prevents the formation of a Morel–Lavallée discharge or seroma.
4. It ensures lymphostasis, although this has not really been proved yet.
5. It reduces traction on the suture line, making the healing process faster and the scar of better quality.
6. It eliminates the need for drainage, since it will be almost impossible to remove a drain because of the glue.

SURGICAL TECHNIQUE

It should be stressed that this operation is intended for moderate fatty-cutaneous lesions. It should be performed under general anaesthesia in a clinic or a hospital, with a hospitalization of 2–4 days.

Preparation

The horseshoe incision/excision is marked on the patient in the upright position. The superior line follows the outline of the pubic hair and forms an equilateral triangle, each side measuring 7 cm (see Fig. 10.9).

The direction of the tunnels is marked using the criss-crossing method and locating on the patient, in the upright position, the areas of maximal fat deposit.

Infiltration is via the wet method (see Chapter 9). The whole abdominal wall is infiltrated, injecting every 5 cm with a 5-cm needle perpendicularly to the abdominal wall, avoiding the 1 cm of superficial subcutaneous fat that will be kept. Up to 500 cm³ of physiological saline can be injected. A 15 minute wait is necessary for hydrodissection to take place and for adrenalin to react.

The operation

Initial supraumbilical liposuction

If this is necessary, its approach is intraumbilical. Great care is needed in this area, limited upward by the xiphoid and laterally by the ribs, where the midline always forms a vertical depression (Fig. 10.10)

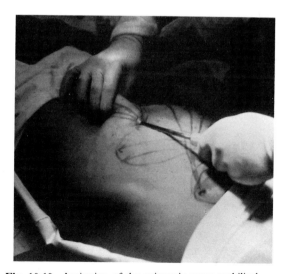

Fig. 10.10 Aspiration of the epigastric supra-umbilical area from an umbilical approach.

It has already been seen that the deep fat that will be aspirated is structurally different from the subumbilical fat.

Initial subumbilical liposuction (Fig. 10.11)

This is done from two small lateral pubic incisions located in the horseshoe zone. These disappear with the first piece resected.

A right-handed operator uses his left hand to grasp the panniculus between the thumb and the other four fingers. The tunnels are started from two 5 mm long incisions, located in the pubic area, with Metzenbaum scissors. First the 8 mm cannula is used and then the 6 mm and 4 mm ones.

Liposuction is carried out in a fanshape and following different planes. The upper layer of fatty tissue, above the superficial fascia, should constantly be checked with the roll test and the pinch test to make sure that the cannulas are always at a depth of at least 1 cm. Perforation of the muscular abdominal wall, although it does happen, is unthinkable to the authors.

The procedure should be slow and regular. If an atraumatic technique is followed with the use of adrenalin, the result should be almost pure fat in the suction bottle. As soon as blood is seen on the cannula or in the transparent hose, the operator should change to another tunnel.

Fluid replacement by the use of macromolecules is indispensable. After liposuction of the epigastric and subumbilical areas, the actual surgery can begin.

Initial in-hair pubic incision/excision

This is horseshoe-shaped, as already described. The equilateral triangle (each side measuring 7 cm) with its inferior apex will return to a normal size at the end of the operation (each side measuring 11–12 cm) after being distended by the tension of the superior flap (Fig. 10.12).

Dissection of the subumbilical stage

This should be moderate, and should not go beyond the suction tunnels that the operator can

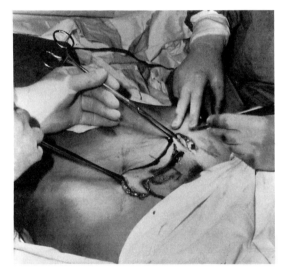

Fig. 10.12 In-hair pubic incision/excision, removing the two approaches of the sub-umbilical liposuction.

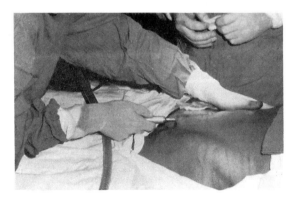

Fig. 10.11 Sub-umbilical aspiration using the crossed tunnels method from two intrapubic mini-incisions.

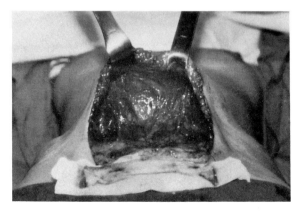

Fig. 10.13 Dissection allowing verification of the evenness of the lipo-suction and the haemostasis and enabling umbilical disinsertion if necessary.

see perfectly, along with the intact perforating arteries, veins and nerves (Fig. 10.13). The dissection of the superior flap should be carried out as required, as in face-lifting, with no undermining limits, the goal being to restore the subumbilical stage to normal tension. This dissection allows:

1. The preservation of most of the vessels undamaged by liposuction;
2. Checking of the even thickness of the remaining fatty panniculus;
3. Completion of the lipectomy surgically with Metzenbaum scissors if asymmetry does exist;
4. Completion of haemostasis of the perforating arteries;
5. Treatment of any musculoaponeurotic lesions, as seen in Chapter 8.

This dissection can be extended to the umbilicus if required.

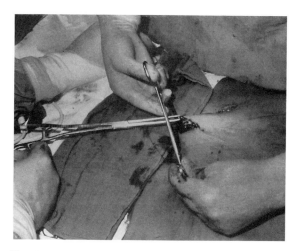

Fig. 10.14 Crossing the flaps.

Umbilical disinsertion

Without a dissection of the subumbilical stage this permits the closure of the aponeurotic breach corresponding to the old umbilicus; it allows the umbilicus to slide down by no more than 2–3 cm; and the umbilicus to be fixed with a non-absorbable thread to the linea alba.

Secondary cutaneous resection (Fig. 10.14)

Using two forceps (Museux, Kocher or Martel), the inferior flap is lowered all the way to the upper side of the pubic triangle. The excess is cut along the midline and staystitched without tightening. The two excess lateral flaps are resected either by pulling downwards only, or downwards and inwards, criss-crossing the flaps and reducing the size of the scar, or downwards and outwards, increasing the size of the scars but allowing a better redraping.

After this secondary resection there is a major loss of substance: usually 7 cm in height and 20 cm in width. Two staystitches are placed, each from one angle of the remaining pubic triangle to the superior flap (Fig. 10.15).

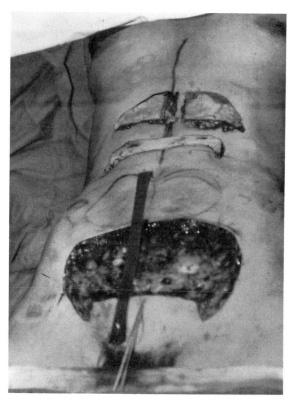

Fig. 10.15 Second cutaneous resection: the substance loss is important. Traction of the upper flap end of the remaining pubic triangle, we obtain: a pubic triangle of normal size (10–12 cm × 10–12 cm); an umbilical pubic triangle distance of 13 cm approximately.

Use of fibrin glue (Fig. 10.16)

The median and the two lateral staystitches are left loose and the thread is held with a forceps. The flap is lifted with two Gillies hooks, and the fibrin glue is sprayed on, using pressurized oxygen, 0.5 cm³ for each 10 × 10 cm quadrilateral (Fig. 10.17). Between 2 and 4 cm³ are needed to completely glue a subumbilical stage.

Immediately after spraying, and while the assistant ties up the staystitches, the surgeon pulls on the subumbilical abdominal skin and brings its inferior side all the way to the superior side of the pubic triangle, holding it steady for 3 minutes (Fig. 10.18).

The sutures

These start at each end of the horizontal scar. The authors prefer to use surgical clips (Cricket, Autosuture), as they leave a better scar. They are quick and easy to handle and can be moved around without a problem if necessary (Fig. 10.19). The staystitches should be replaced by buried absorbable sutures (Maxon).

As for the lateral ends of the scar, there are three possibilities:

1. By 'cheating' a little, the lateral sides of the pubic triangle can be sutured using surgical thread or clips: the final scar will be horseshoe-shaped and entirely hidden by the pubic hair.

2. Liposuction can reduce the extent of any lateral 'dog ears'. The cutaneous portion can be corrected using the 'inverted triangles' method and turning down the ears on either side of the pubic triangle. This will result in a 'minilift'-type suture (Glicenstein).

3. The 'ears' could also be transversely resected. The final suture line will be completely horizontal, and will be three-quarters hidden by the pubic hair.

One of the advantages of liposuction is in the correction of the thickness incongruity between the two edges.

The absence of tension, due to the 'as required' resection, as in face-lifting, and to the use of fibrin glue, relieves the suture and avoids the formation of buried scars. These are usually due to the fibrous adhesion of the skin to the deep aponeurotic plane, without subcutaneous fat but with fatty tissue above and below the scar. This is how these unattractive scars form.

It is not advisable to use any kind of vacuum drainage in the presence of fibrin glue, since there is no deadspace left and the extraction of the drain tubes would be extremely difficult.

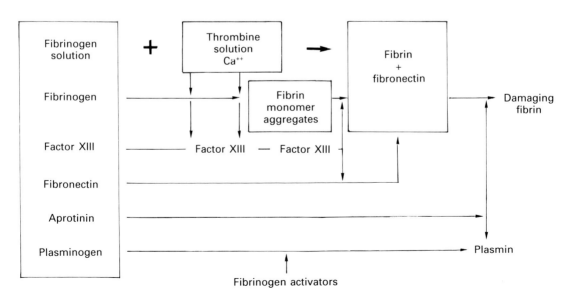

Fig. 10.16 Combination of two components: fibrinogen and thrombin.

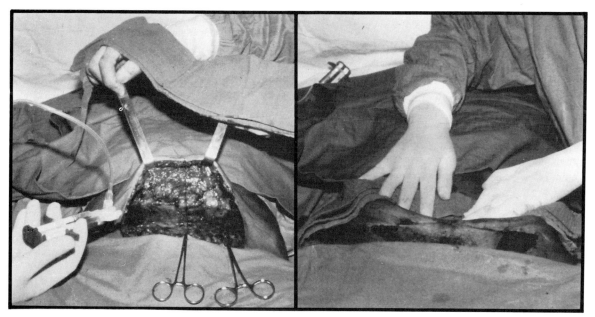

Fig. 10.17 Spraying the glue. Notice the shine of the glue.

Fig. 10.18 'The art of glueing'.

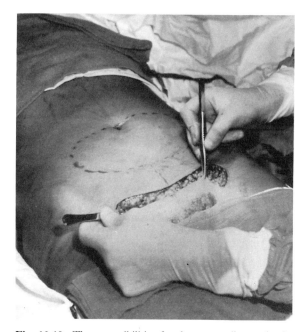

Fig. 10.19 Three possibilities for the suture: 'horse shoe'; horizontal low transverse; mini-lift.

The dressing is simple: the suture line is covered with gauze and supra- and subumbilical absorbent pads are placed on top. The patient should immediately wear the 'lipo-panty' mentioned earlier.

Postoperative care

This is simple, with a first check after 48 hours. Ecchymoses are frequent. Major haematomas are rare, but require prompt evacuation if they occur.

As early as the second day, if the patient leans forward she will notice that the abdominal skin adheres to the deep layer.

The sutures and clips are removed in two sessions, no later than the 10th day, since the use of fibrin glue eliminates any tension. Pressotherapy and lymphatic drainage will be started on the 15th day by a physiotherapist to be continued for 1 month.

The patient should wear the lipo-panty day and night for the first month, and 12 hours a day for the following 15 days. She should be warned that she will not really notice the final result before the end of the second month.

Potential complications of liposuction and the surgery will be discussed in detail in Chapter 11.

CONCLUSION

A low localized abdominoplasty has been proposed for moderate fatty-cutaneous lesions. This will be combined with primary liposuction, always subumbilical and seldom supraumbilical, with or without umbilical disinsertion, and using a fibrin glue to eliminate any detachment at the end of the operation.

This operation, that the authors have called cosmetic suction abdominoplasty or CSA, and that has been reported at the meeting of the International Society of Plastic and Reconstructive Surgery (New Delhi, March 1987), and to the Société Française de Chirurgie Plastique Reconstructive et Esthétique (Hammamet, June 1987), and published in *Annales de Chirurgie Plastique* (N° 2, 1987), is starting to give some very satisfactory cosmetic results. Only 10 years ago, these patients would have been refused surgery, because the classic low transverse scar appeared to be too gross for such moderate lesions.

11. Potential complications

The patient should be warned about these possible and frequent complications at the first consultation. This chapter will consider the complications of abdominoplasty without liposuction. Grazer's (1975) study of 10 490 patients and 945 operators from the *American Society of Plastic and Reconstructive Surgeons* represents a unique reference series. The complications of an isolated abdominal liposuction, and of abdominoplasty associated with liposuction will also be discussed.

ABDOMINOPLASTY WITHOUT LIPOSUCTION

Mortality

Like any other surgical procedure, abdominoplasty has a mortality rate, which is currently 17/10 490 or 1.6/1000. This disturbing rate should be considered objectively, bearing in mind that there are many different surgical procedures under the name abdominoplasty, ranging from localized abdominoplasty with no umbilical procedure in the young patient, to a three-quarter lipectomy for a pendulous abdomen in the obese patient.

Thromboembolic accidents

These are phlebitis (1.1%), pulmonary embolism (0.8%) and death (0.5%). This is a serious risk, as in all abdominal surgery. The phlebitis rate is probably lower than the actual one since a study using marked fibrinogen showed a rate of 7% in gynaecological operations using a vaginal approach. This complication presents both a therapeutic and a preventive problem.

From a therapeutic point of view, and in the presence of a calf pain that is usually of postural origin, the plastic surgeon is caught in the dilemma of uncontrollable haematoma due to anticoagulant therapy, and thromboembolic panic. The authors' approach is as follows: no previous anticoagulant therapy, careful clinical evaluation, echography and Doppler examination if necessary; angiography if phlebitis is suspected and heparinotherapy if the diagnosis is confirmed.

Prevention consists of a number of rules and suggestions, none of which is 100% certain:

1. Refuse surgery to all high-risk patients who might have thromboembolic problems.
2. Avoid compression of the popliteal area during the operation.
3. Some authors suggest massaging the calf area during the operation.
4. The operating time should be reduced to a minimum.
5. Some mention the intraabdominal hypertension due to excessive tension on the superior flap or the musculoaponeurotic layer.
6. Early ambulation is essential.
7. Many studies suggest that the contraceptive pill could be responsible for thromboembolic accidents. The patient should be advised to stop taking the pill a month before surgery.

Haematoma

This has an incidence of 6%. If it occurs before the 15th day, the haematoma could become a factor in infection and necrosis. A fibrous organization will occur and for the next 6 months to a year the abdominal wall will look asymmetrical and indurated, resembling orange peel, and very unsightly. Treatment depends on its size: for a small haematoma, prompt evacuation and puncture; for a large haematoma, reoperation is necessary.

For this particular operation, haemostasis must be meticulous, tying rather than coagulating the deep segment of the perforating arteries before they retract, and checking haemostasis before closing the wound. Good drainage, using one or two drains, helps evacuate any discharge.

The use of biological glues, based on human fibrinogen and bovine thrombin, eliminates any deadspace. In this case drainage cannot be used and good haemostasis is still mandatory: the absence of drainage could be catastrophic with poor haemostasis. Finally there is the possibility of a haematoma located directly behind the abdominal wall, that could have very serious complications. In some cases the compression due to the dressing helps prevent haematomas, but if this compression is too great it could cause necrosis of the flap.

Morel–Lavallée discharge (SEROMA)

This is a seroma as described by Morel–Lavallée in 1853. It contains a clear liquid, very rich in albumin and containing both fatty and red blood cells. The author called it a 'serous discharge'. According to Morel–Lavallée, the mechanism consists of a serous oozing through ruptured small capillary vessels. It cannot be coagulated and is not of lymphatic origin.

Clinically, the picture is as follows: as soon as the drains are removed (around the 7th day), the drainage will be a clear yellow fluid and the abdomen will begin to swell. As early as the 10th day a discharge is visible, and palpation of the abdominal wall produces a fluid wave. Aspiration with the patient in the lateral decubitus position drains out a clear liquid (50–150 ml). Such aspiration performed under sterile conditions every 3 days shows that the quantity of fluid decreases with time and disappears after 1 month.

A thin layer of fat on the musculoaponeurotic plane will not prevent this complication from happening, but the use of biological glues could be an effective prevention, essentially because they eliminate any deadspace.

This discharge is common after an isolated liposuction. This is why pressotherapy and elastic compression are important and should be started by a physiotherapist no later than 10 days after the operation.

Necrosis

Necrosis is a rare occurrence, but according to Grazer's study, 40% of all surgeons have had at least one case of necrosis; the obverse is that 60% have not. Those that have been referred to the authors from elsewhere have usually been consequent on lipectomy in obese patients and in three-branch suture lines.

The site of necrosis is almost always the superior edge, corresponding to the old supra-umbilical area. It is usually very small but could reach several centimetres. The occasional rare necrosis of the entire flap can only be due to a very serious technical error, or to gas gangrene.

Studies on abdominal blood supply show distribution to be in the shape of a three-branched candelabra, and indicate that it is not easy to cause an arterially induced necrosis unless the cleft is very superficial or there is an anomalous blood supply. However, studies of the venous system demonstrate that morbidity or necrosis of a portion of the flap is more logically connected with the obstruction of venous return.

In the event of such necrosis occurring, it is best to excise it surgically. This is an insensitive area so no anaesthesia is required. The contraction of the excision edges will considerably reduce the defect, and a cosmetic 'touch up', if required by the patient, could be done 6 months later. A skin graft would emphasize the defect itself but might be indicated in the case of serious and extensive necrosis.

The principles of prevention are as follows:

1. Avoid excessive traction on the superior flap, and do not always perform a low transverse abdominoplasty with umbilical transposition, simply out of habit.
2. Limit the detachment as much as possible

in the obese patient and never go beyond the floating ribs and the xiphoid.

3. Prevent the onset of a haematoma by excellent haemostasis.

4. Do not perform lipectomy of the deep side of the superior flap with a scalpel. Liposuction has made this procedure obsolete.

5. Make sure that there is good vascularization of the flaps and help it, if necessary, with flexion of the thighs.

6. In the presence of previous abdominal scars, great care must be taken before abdominoplasty (if the excision will not remove the scar). Some precautions are necessary:

- A minimum of 1 year is required for the necessary recanalization and revascularization before abdominoplasty;
- Preserve an undetached area around the scar in order to save the underlying perforating arteries;
- If the scar is too long or the arterial terrain uncertain, do not perform any surgery;
- Ask the heavy smoker to stop smoking for a month before and after surgery. Limit the detachment and the traction on the superior flap.

Umbilical necrosis is exceptional, especially if the fatty tissue around the transposed umbilicus is maintained.

Infection

Infection is a rare occurrence but the possibility is greater in the face of blood or lymph discharge and necrosis. The risk is even higher with an obese patient, skin lesions around the folds (pendulous abdomen), injured peritoneum and increased operative time. It could be very serious in the obese patient and some cases of gas gangrene have been reported. The treatment is surgical followed by an antibiotic therapy according to the bacteria present.

To prevent infection it is necessary to maintain rigorous asepsis, to keep on washing the surgical field during the operation, to reduce the operating time and to treat any skin lesions several weeks before the operation. It is also necessary to keep

the detachment minimal in the obese patient. The use of prophylactic antibiotics during and after the operation should be limited to the high-risk patient. Although infection is rare, it is very damaging to the final result.

Problems with reinnervation

On the day following a low transverse abdominoplasty, it is normal enough for the patient to feel the fingers of the surgeon on the floating ribs; as the palpation moves downwards there is an increase in numbness as far as the pubic area, where it is complete. In studying the innervation of the abdominal wall, it is readily seen that there is total interruption of the sensory innervation because of the incision and the undermining of the superior flap. Full sensation returns after 6–8 months. The patient must be warned of this numbness, if only to prevent hot-water bottle burns, for example, as the authors have seen in one patient.

Residual problems and defects (Fig. 11.1)

The scar

If subcuticular continuous or half-buried horizontal mattress sutures are used, with the knot always on the pubic side, and if the sutures are removed early enough, the scar will at best be acceptable on the 15th day. It will need a 2-minute manual massage in the morning and evening daily for 2 months. This can be done by the patient herself. The scar should not be exposed to sunlight during the first year.

The scar will be red and raised at the end of the second month. One to three injections of corticosteroid directly into the scar may then be necessary.

At the end of the first year the scar may still be red, wide, and quite visible. It may have adhesions to the deep plane, especially after a Morel–Lavallée discharge. Its appearance will be much better after 2–3 years, and will age very well.

More seriously, it could develop into a true keloid scar, especially in hair-bearing areas and in black or yellow skin. This is a totally different

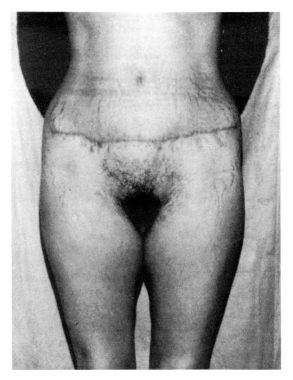 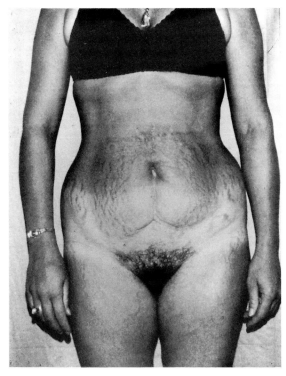

Fig. 11.1 a and b Residual problems and defects: **a** irregular, asymetrical and raised scar; **b** poor indication and poor result.

study, and cannot be included in this book. The authors simply note that the scar will look acceptable relatively quickly in obese patients and after vertical plasty.

Topography

The raising of the inferior edge provokes a distension of the pubic triangle and is due to an excessive traction of the superior flap (dyspareunia has even been reported). Usually this is because the indications for low transverse abdominoplasty with umbilical transposition were poor, and excessive traction was necessary to lower the supraumbilical flap down to the pubis. This difficulty is encountered with a long wrinkled abdomen: in such cases it is better to perform a low transverse abdominoplasty without umbilical transposition but with umbilical disinsertion.

An asymmetry of the scar is not uncommon

and a procedure to limit this defect has been described.

The scar is much easier to hide if it is short, low and causes no distension of the pubic triangle, i.e. resulting from localized plasties focused on the pubic triangle and adapted to the lesions. This means that vertical plasties should be reserved for existing scars and low plasties should be well indicated to avoid the raising of the lower edge, as has already been seen.

Redraped skin

Insufficient redraping can be global, with the recurrence of ptosis, or lateral with a persistence of 'dog ears'. It usually results from the desire to keep the scar as short as possible, thus reducing the lateral skin excision.

Excessive skin requires a raising of the lower flap. In the case of stretchmarked and wrinkled skin, a spreading of the superior flap is necessary in order to redrape the skin. The process of gathering the flap so as to balance the two edges should be avoided.

ISOLATED LIPOSUCTION

Some complications are inherent to liposuction as others are to abdominoplasty.

Complications

Abdominal perforation

This is an exceptional complication and of course extremely serious. It can be avoided by rigorous technique and blunt cannulas and by staying away from parietal weakness points (hernias, eventration, laparotomy scar).

Fluid and electrolyte imbalance, haematocrit changes.

These occur if the aspirated volume exceeds 1.5 litres. The entire volume should be replaced by liquid substitution during and after the operation.

Haematoma, infection and lymphatic discharge

These can occur even with rigorous asepsis and immediate elastic compression.

Postoperative ecchymoses are a common occurrence and disappear after 2–3 weeks.

Oedema. The onset is fast and masks the result, but it disappears after 1–2 months. Compression speeds up its resorption.

Defects

There are three main defects:

Residual skin excess

This takes the form of a 'wave'. The excess is due to the inability of the skin to redrape itself over the new subcutaneous volume, and to an incorrect preoperative assessment of the retractile power of the skin; the procedure for correct assessment has been explained in an earlier chapter. This excess could be treated with secondary cutaneous reduction plasty.

Fatty unevenness

This is due to an uneven liposuction technique that leaves behind some fatty islets. It can be differentiated from skin excess by the following test: if the patient is in a reclining position, the condition due to skin excess disappears and the one due to an uneven procedure persists. This defect could be treated with additional liposuction under local anaesthesia.

Subcutaneous damage

This is due to the removal of superficial subcutaneous fatty tissue by a poor handling of the liposuction cannula, directed superficially with an upward suction. Treatment is difficult and consists of the reinjection of aspirated fat. However, this method is still very controversial, although it is widely used. These defects are not specific to abdominal liposuction but in this area they are very visible to the patient.

ASSOCIATION OF LIPOSUCTION WITH ABDOMINOPLASTY

This association adds no complications to those already described. However it seems to the authors that there is a greater incidence of Morel–Lavallée discharge. Its prevention is difficult but could be facilitated by suprapubic drainage for a period of 3 weeks. It is effective but constraining. The use of fibrin glue seems to be promising.

12. Indications and results

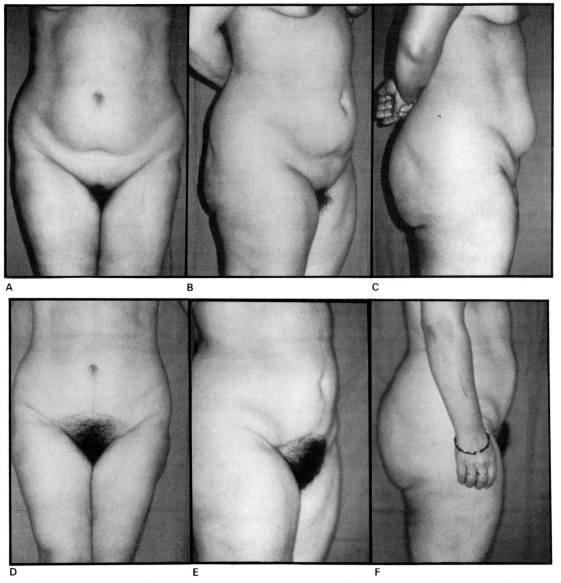

Fig. 12.1 Low transverse abdominal dermolipectomy without any umbilical procedure, (patient of Figs 8.60, 8.61, and 8.62.) **a, b and c**: pre-operative state. **d, e, and f**: result, 1 year later.

Fig. 12.2

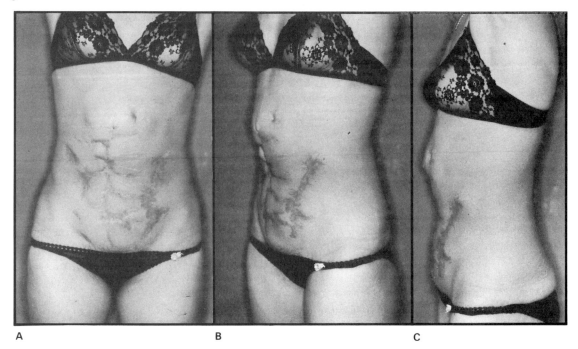

A   B   C

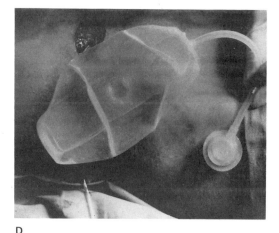

D

The different indications have been discussed at length in Chapters 3 and 8, with the different clinical pictures and operative techniques. It should be remembered that from a 'mono-morphous' operation, consisting most of the time of a low transverse lipectomy with umbilical transposition, plastic surgery of the abdomen has become a 'polymorphous' operation, allowing the

treatment of various problems, often less major than in the past, with more suitable techniques. This is the principle behind the new edition of this book.

OBJECTIVES

In order to achieve the objective of plastic surgery, certain requirements concerning indications, technique and surgical care should be borne in mind.

The indication should be adapted to the particular lesion and make the treatment of the muscular fatty-cutaneous defects possible with an acceptable scar. The choice will actually be between the various disadvantages.

The appropriate technique should lead to the different cosmetic goals:

1. To eliminate any skin excess. The redraping of the skin should be sufficient to eliminate as many skin lesions as possible, but not so excessive as to cause deformation of the pubic triangle or any distension of the scar.

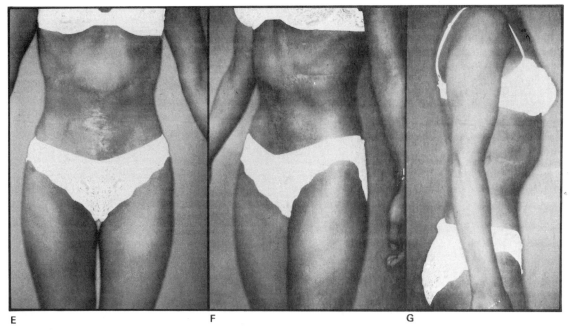

E   F   G

Fig. 12.2 Multiple scars from peritonitis (patient of Fig. 3.2). Treatment with skin expansion, (using two lateral expandors). **a, b and c**: preoperative state. **d e, f and g**: result 18 months later.

Fig. 12.3

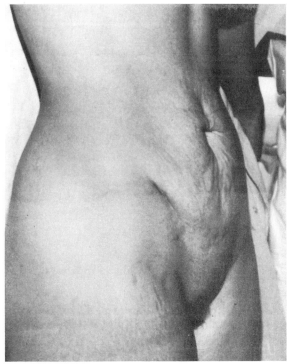

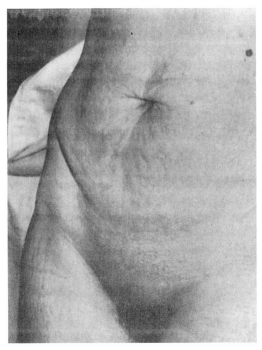

A   B

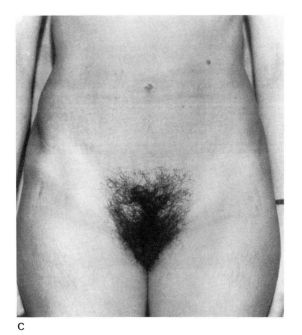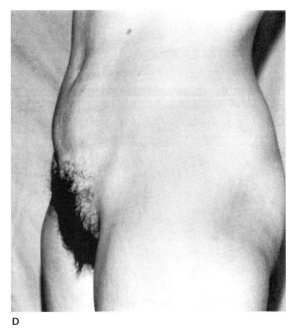

C   D

Fig. 12.3 a and **b** pre-operative state. **c** result of transverse plasty, 2 years later (frontal view). **d** same patient 2 years later (three-quarter view).

2. To eliminate any possible adipose excess.
3. To treat any diastasis of the rectus abdominis.
4. To leave the best possible scar, that is easy to conceal: this is a main element of the final result.

As far as surgical care is concerned, abdominoplasty could be very helpful for many patients. Its success depends on the right indications and technique, but also on the thorough information, given by the surgeon, regarding the difficulties, the hazards, the limitations of the procedure, and the resulting scar. The location of the future scar should be demonstrated and the patient warned of the necessary patience needed before the scar becomes acceptable.

INDICATIONS

There are four major clinical and anatomical indications.

The obese patient

This is a combination of skin excess and abdominal fat excess that extends laterally. A classic three-quarter lipectomy with umbilical transposition will treat the cutaneous distension but not the corresponding adipose excess. An associated liposuction, performed first during the same operation, will be an indispensable complementary procedure, as it eliminates the adipose excess of the abdominal wall and the lateral extensions; it reduces the thickness incongruity of the edges, facilitating the suture and improving the scar; it also replaces all indications for circular lipectomy (Fig. 12.1).

Post-pregnancy dermal dystrophy

This is an indication for a classic abdominoplasty without liposuction. The resection should be adapted to the lesions and the scar should be the smallest possible.

A low transverse abdominoplasty with umbilical transposition is not the only therapeutic possibility. In some cases, a mixed vertical and transverse abdominoplasty could be used, or a vertical procedure or even just a localized mid-abdominal one (Figs 12.2, 12.3).

Moderate fatty-cutaneous lesions of the abdominal wall

For these moderate lesions consisting simply of an average increase in the adipose panniculus and

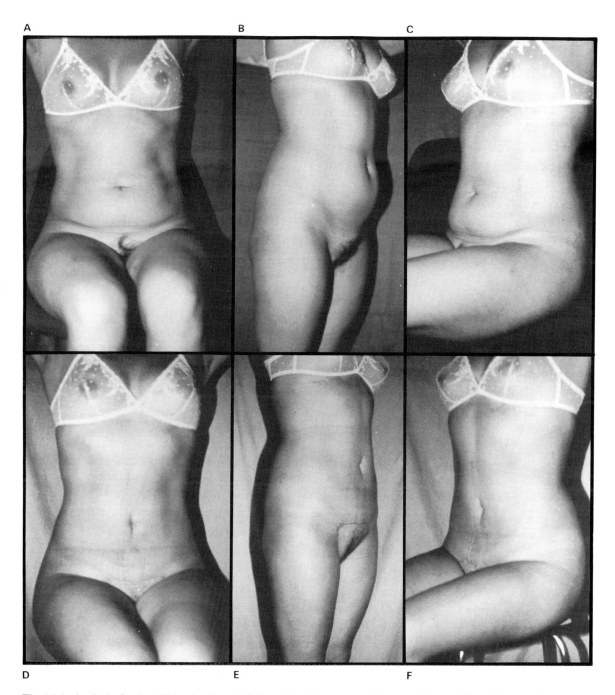

Fig. 12.4 Aesthetic Suction Abdominoplasty (ASA). **a, b and c**: preoperative state. **d, e and f**: result 1 year later.

a slight cutaneous distension, a low localized abdominoplasty can be used, that combines:

1. Liposuction, subumbilical and possibly supraumbilical;
2. A low transverse fusiform cutaneous resection, the lower edge being in the pubic triangle;
3. A possible disinsertion–lowering of the umbilicus, without transposition;
4. A redraping of the upper abdominal flap and possible additional resection of the residual cutaneous excess.
5. The use of fibrin glue.

The authors have obtained some very satisfactory results with this operation in many patients suffering from moderate fatty-cutaneous lesions of the abdominal wall. It has been called aesthetic suction abdominoplasty, or ASA (Fig. 12.4).

Small or average abdominal fat excess without cutaneous excess

The adipose excess is usually in the subumbilical area. Most of the time, the skin is healthy and quite tonic. With liposuction, there is now something to offer these patients: an isolated abdominal liposuction without cutaneous reduction plasty will treat this defect, leaving no scar. With good indications and a rigorous technique, the results are excellent (Fig. 12.5).

CONCLUSION

It is difficult to assess the value of the authors' results since the introduction of these techniques and the association of the different procedures are quite recent. This modern approach is added to the usual reasons that have always made difficult any analysis of the results of abdominoplasty, in that it is necessary to wait 2–3 years; it is difficult to judge one's own results with total objectivity; and the result is partly subjective. Nevertheless, it seems that three points should be emphasized:

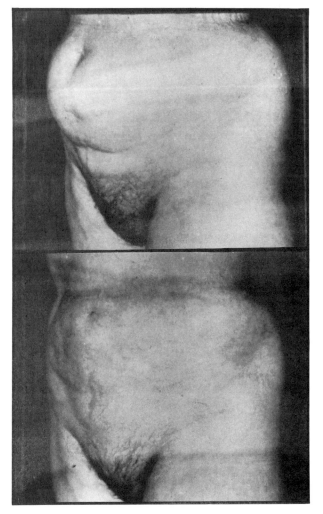

Fig. 12.5 Isolated abdominal liposuction for moderate abdominal fat excess: **a** preoperative state; **b** result 6 months later.

1. Excellent cosmetic results can now be obtained with plastic surgery of the abdomen. Only 10 years ago, this was not the case.
2. Abdominoplasty is a procedure that ages quite well: the surgeon is usually pleasantly surprised to see his results after 3 years.
3. The plastic surgeon has an 'obligation of modesty' when dealing with abdominoplasty.

Bibliography

Agris J. — Apparatus to hold panniculus up during abdominoplasty. *Plast. Reconstr. Surg.*, *60*, 2, 292–3, 1977.

Allansmith R. — An excision of abdominal fat apron. *A. M. A. Arch. Surg.*, *80*, 327, 1960.

Apfelberg D. B. et coll. — Two unusual umbilicoplasties. *Plast. Reconstr. Surg.*, *64*, 2, 268–70, 1979.

Appiani E. — Muscular plastic for aesthetic conformation of abdominal girdle. *Ann. Plast. Surg.*, *13*, 2, 97–106, 1984.

Ashbell T. S. — Abdominoplasty and combined procedure (letter). *Plast. Reconstr. Surg.*, *79*, 2, 316, 1987.

Avelar J. M. — Abdominoplasty: methodization of a technique without external umbilical scar. *Aesth. Plast. Surg.*, *2*, 141–151, 1978.

Avelar J. M. — Fat suction versus abdominoplasty. *Aesth. Plast. Surg.*, *2*, 4, 265–75, 1985.

Avelar J. M. — Abdominoplasty: technical refinement and analysis of 130 cases in 8 years follow-up. *Aesth. Plast. Surg.*, *7*, 4, 205–12, 1983.

Avelar J. M. — Study of the anatomy of the subcutaneous adipose tissue applied for fat suction technique. *Travail de l'Institut Scientifique Brésilien de Chirurgie Plastique*, Sao Paulo, 1986.

Babcock W. W. — The correction of the obese and relaxed abdominal wall with special reference to the used of buried siver charm. *Am. J. Obstet.*, *596*, 1916, 1974.

Bailey A. J., Robins S. P. — Development and maturation of the crosslinks in the collagen fibers of skin. *In: Aging of connective tissues*, pp. 130–156. Karger, Bâle, 1973.

Baran N. K., Celebi C. — A ten-year experience with reduction mammaplasty and abdominoplasty. What is happening in our part of the world? *Clin. Plast. Surg.*, *11*, 3, 479–89, 1984.

Barett B. M., Kelly M. V. — Combined abdominoplasty and augmentation mammaplasty through a transverse suprapubic incision. *Ann. Plast. Surg.*, *4*, 4, 286–91, 1980.

Baroudi R. et coll. — Abdominoplasty. *Plast. Reconstr. Surg.*, *54*, 2, 161–167, 1974.

Baroudi R., Keppke E. M., Carvalho C. G. — Mammary reduction combined with reverse abdominoplasty. *Ann. Plast, Surg*, *2*, 5, 368–73, 1979.

Barraya L., Napkane E. — Abdomen molluscum. Abdomen pendulum. Réparation. Nouvel ombilic. *Presse Méd.*, *48–76*, 2287, 1968.

Barsky A. S., Kahn S. — *Principles and practice of plastic surgery*. Mc Graw Hill, New York, 1964.

Berlan M., Lafontan M. — Les alpha-2 récepteurs. *Quotidien du Médecin*, *19*, suppl. n° 2855, 35–40, 1983.

Biesenberger H. — Abdomen pendulous. *Zbl. chir.*, *63*, 1399, 1936.

Bjornstorp. — Human adipose tissue. Dynamic and regulation. *Metabolic Disease*, *5*, 277, 1971.

Bostwick J. et coll. — Blood supply of the abdomen revisited, with emphasis on the superficial inferior epigastric artery. *Plast. Reconstr. Surg.*, *74*, 5, 657–70, 1984.

Bostwick J., Hill H. L., Nahai F. — Repairs in the lower abdomen, groin, or perineum with myocutaneous or omental flaps. *Plast. Reconstr. Surg.*, *63*, 2, 186–94, 1979.

Bouissou H., Pieraggi M. T., Julian M., Douste Blazy L. — Cutaneous aging. Its relation with arteriosclerosis and atheroma. *In: Aging of connective tissues*, pp. 199–211. Karger, Bâle, 1973.

Boyd J., Taylor G., Corlett R. — The vascular territories of the superieur and the deep inferior epigastric systems. *Plast. Reconstr. Surg.*, *73*, 1, 1–16, 1984.

Brodeur A., Charbonneau R. — Grossesse et chirurgie esthétique. *Union, Med. Can.*, *113*, 3, 169–71, 1984.

Callia W. — Contribuicão para o estudo da correção cirurgica do abdome penduloe globoso. Técnica original. *Thèse mèd.*, São Paulo, 1965.

Callia W. E. P. — Una plastica para à cirugiao geral. *Medecina hospitalar*, *1*, 40–41, 1967.

Caravel J. B. — Plasties abdominales. Technique personnelle de reconstruction ombilicale. Report de la cicatrice au fond de l'ombilic. *Ann. Chir. Plast. Esthét.*, *26*, 3, 289–292, 1981.

Cardoso de Castro C. et coll. — T abdominoplasty to remove multiples scars from the abdomen. *Ann. Plast. Surg.*, *12*, 4, 369–73, 1984.

Cardoso de Castro C., Daher M. — Simultaneous reduction mammaplasty and abdominoplasty. *Plast. Reconstr. Surg.*, *61*, 1, 36–9, 1978.

Carreirao S. et coll. — Treatment of abdominal wall eventrations associated with abdominoplasty techniques. *Aesthet. Plast. Surg.*, *8*, 3, 173–9, 1984.

Castanares S., Goethel J. A. — Abdominal lipectomy, a modification in technique. *Plast. Reconst. Surg.*, *40*, 3, 378–83, 1967.

Champy M., Khouri M., Antz D. — Intérêt clinique d'une nouvelle colle biologique: la *Transglutine*. *Ann. Chir. Plast. Esthét.*, *32*, 2, 178–180, 1987.

Chiu H. W. — Tensor fasciae latae free flap for full-thickness abdominal wall reconstruction utilizing the greater omentum as a vascular supply-letter. *Plast.*

Reconstr. Surg., 75, 4, 607, 1985.

Christman K. D. — Death following suction lipectomy and abdominoplasty. Plast. Reconstr. Surg., 78, 3, 428, 1986.

Clarkson P., Jeef J. — The contribution of plastic surgery to the treatment of obesity. In: Modern trends in plastic surgery, pp. 315–336. Butterworths, London, 1966.

Converse J. M. — Reconstructive plastic surgery. W. B. Saunders, C° Philadelphia, 1977.

Correa Iturraspe M. — Dermolipectomia vertical del abdomen. Bol. Soc. Argent. Ciruj., 13, 648–651, 1952.

Costagliola M. — Abdomen pendulum et éventrations monstrueux. Communication à la Société Française de Chirurgie Plastique. Ajaccio, 1970.

Courtiss E. H. — Suction lipectomy: A retrospective analysis of 100 patients. Plast. Reconstr. Surg., 73, 5, 780–794, 1984.

Davis T. S. — Morbid obesity. Clin. Plast. Surg., 11, 3, 517–524, 1984.

Debaere P. A. — Chirurgie morphologique abdominale. Thèse de doctorat, Lille, 1975.

Debaere P. A. — Psychologie de l'obèse, candidat à la lipectomie. Thèse de doctorat, Lille, 1975.

Dellon A. L. — Fleur de lis abdominoplasty. Aesthet. Plast. Surg., 9, 1, 27–32, 1985.

Depaulis J. — La chirurgie des abdomens pendulums. Réflexions sur 20 cas. J. Méd. Bordeaux, 144, 5, 697–712, 1967.

Derouinaud A. — Les plasties abdominales. Thèse Méd., Toulouse, 1973.

Detrie P. — L'opéré abdominal. Masson, Paris, 1970.

Devernois de Bonnefon J. F. — Chirurgie du ventre en tablier, par incision en « T » renversé. Concours Méd., 78, 22, 2587–2589, 1956.

Dubou R., Ousterhout D. K. — Placement of the umbilicus in an abdominoplasty. Plast. Reconstr. Surg., 61, 2, 291–298, 1978.

Dufourmentel C., Mouly R. — Chirurgie plastique. Collection médico-chirurgicale. Flammarion, Paris, 1959.

Elbaz J. S. — A propos des plasties abdominales. Technique du « fer à cheval ». Ann. Chir. Plast., 19, 2, 155–158, 1974.

Elbaz J. S., Flageul G. — Plastic surgery of the abdomen. Masson, New York, 1978.

Elbaz J. S., Flageul G. — Chirurgie plastique de l'abdomen. Masson, Paris, 1978.

Elbaz J. S. — Abdominoplastie à visée esthétique avec liposuccion première. Ann. Chir. Plast. Esthét., 32, 2, 148–151, 1987.

Elbaz J. S. — Les plasties abdominales. Immex Spécial Annuel, 711–721, 1972.

Elbaz J. S. — Pannel des abdominoplasties. V° Congrès de l'IPRS, Paris, 1975.

Elbaz J. S., Dardour J.C., Ricbourg B. — Vascularisation artérielle de la paroi abdominale. Ann. Chir. Plast., 20, 1, 19–29, 1975.

Elbaz J. S., Flageul G. — Liposuccion isolée et liposuccion-plastie. Congrès SFCPRE, Bruxelles, mai 1986.

Elbaz J. S., Flageul G., Sitbon E. — Abdominoplasty. 1/ The epic. 2/ The conquest. International Congress of Plastic and Aesthetic Surgery, New Dehli, 1987.

Elbaz J. S., Zumer L. — Maternité et préjudices esthétiques. Les dossiers de l'Obstétrique, 2, 16–22, 1974.

Elsahy N. — Abdominoplasty combined with correction of the flaccidity of the lateral lower abdomen and the flanks. Aesthet. Plast. Surg., 9, 1, 33–7, 1985.

Faivre J. — La chirurgie esthétique et le médecin praticien. Gazette des Hôpitaux, 23, 55, 1972.

Faivre J. — Chirurgie esthétique de l'abdomen. Maloine, Paris. 1978.

Faivre J. — Chirurgie esthétique. Abdomen et liposuccion. Maloine, Paris, 1986.

Fischer A., Fischer G. M. — Revised technique for cellulitis fat reduction in riding breeches deformity. Bull. Int. Acad. Cosmt. Surg., 2, 40, 1977.

Fischi R. A. — Vertical abdominoplasty. Plast. Reconstr. Surg., 51, 139–143, 1973.

Flageul G., Elbaz J. S. — Les plasties abdominales: analyses des résultats. Congrès SFCPRE, Bruxelles, mai 1986.

Flageul G., Sitbon E. — Pour une correction numérisée de l'incongruence de longueur des berges dans les plasties abdominales transversales. Ann. Chir. Plast. Esthét., 32, 3, 223–226, 1987.

Flesh-Thebesius J., Weinschelner L. — Die Operation des Hängebauches. Chirurg., 3, 841, 1931.

Fomon S. — Cosmetic surgery, principles and practice. J. B. Lippincott C°, Philadelphia, 1960.

Fournier F., Otteni M. — Plasties abdominales hier et aujourd'hui. Dermolipectomies et collapso-chirurgie. (techniques isolées ou associées et progrès récents). Cah. Chir., 50, 2, 11–30, 1984.

Freeman B. S., Weimer D. R. — Abdominoplasty with special emphasis attention to the construction of the umbilicus. Technic and complications. Aesthet. Plast. Surg., 2, 65–74, 1978.

Galtier M. — Traitement chirurgical de l'obésité de la paroi abdominale avec ptose. Mém. Acad. Chir., 81, 341–344, 1955.

Ger R., Duboys E. — The prevention and repair of large abdominal-wall defects by muscle transposition: a preliminary communication. Plast. Reconstr. Surg., 72, 2, 170–8, 1983.

Gillies H., Millard R. — The principles and art of plastic surgery, pp. 291–420, Little Brown and C°, Boston, 1957.

Glicenstein J. — Les difficultés du traitement chirurgical des dermodystrophies abdominales. Ann. Chir. Plast., 20, 2, 147–155, 1975.

Glicenstein J. — Chirurgie esthétique de l'abdomen. La vie Médicale, 2, 27, 3215, 1972.

Goldwyn R. — Abdominoplasty as a combined procedure: Added benefit or double trouble? Plast. Reconstr. Surg., 78, 3, 383–4, 1986.

Gonzales Ulloa M. — Belt lipectomy. Br. J. Plast. Surg., 13, 179–186, 1960.

Gonzales Ulloa M. — Circular lipectomy with transposition of the umbilicus and aponeurolytic technic. Cirur. y Cirur., 27, 394–409, 1959.

Gosset J. — Bandes de peau totale comme matériel de suture autoplastique en chirurgie. Mém. Acad. Chir., 75, 277–279, 1969.

Graham J. K. — Abdominoplasty. J. La State Med. Soc., 135, 7, 11–3, 1983.

Grazer F. M. — Suction-assisted lipectomy. Its indications, contrindications, and complications. In: Habal M. — Advances in plastic and reconstructive surgery, pp. 51–59. Chicago, 1984.

Grazer F. M. — Use of fiber optic bundles in plastic

surgery. *Plast. Reconstr. Surg.*, *48*, 28–31, 1971.

Grazer F. M., Goldwyn R. M. — Abdominoplasty assessed by survey with emphasis on complications. *Plast. Reconstr. Surg.*, *59*, 4, 513–517, 1977.

Grazer F. M. — Suction-assisted lipectomy, suction lipectomy, lipolysis and lipexeresis. *Plast. Reconstr. Surg.*, *72*, 620–623, 1983.

Greminger R. F. — The mini-abdominoplasty. *Plast. Reconstr. Surg.*, *79*, 3, 356–365, 1987

Guerrerosantos J. et coll. — Umbilical reconstruction with secondary abdominoplasty. *Ann. Plast. Surg.*, *5*, 2, 139–144, 1980.

Hakme F. — Abdominoplasty: peri and supra-umbilical lipectomy. *Aesthet. Plast. Surg.*, *7*, 4, 213–220, 1983.

Hayflick L. — Le vieillissement des cellules humaines. *Triangles*, *14*, 2, 129–139, 1974.

Hodgkinson D. J. — Umbilicoplasty: conversion of « outie » to « innie ». *Aesthet. Plast. Surg.*, *7*, 4, 221–222, 1983.

Huger W. E. — The anatomic rationale for abdominal lipectomy. *Am. Surg.*, *45*, 9, 612–617, 1979.

Illouz Y. G. — Remodelage chirurgical de la silhouette par lipolyse-aspiration ou lipectomie selective. *Ann. Chir. Plast. Esthét.*, *29*, 2, 162–179, 1984.

Illouz Y. G. — Les séquelles esthétiques ou les résultats indésirables de la lipoaspiration. *Ann. Chir. Plast. Esthét.*, *32*, 3, 229–245, 1987.

Illouz Y. G. — Une nouvelle technique pour les lipodystrophies. *Communication à la Société Française de Chirurgie Plastique Reconstructrice et Esthétique*, 1978 et 1979.

Illouz Y. G. — Body contouring by liolysis: A 5-year experience with over 3000 cases. *Plast. Reconstr. Surg.*, *72*, 591–597, 1983.

Illouz Y. G. — Une nouvelle technique pour les lipodystrophies localisées. *Rev. Chir. Esthét Langue Fr.*, 6, 19, 1980.

Isaacs G. — Breast shaping procedures, abdominoplasty, and thighplasty in Australia. *Clin. Plast. Surg.*, *11*, 3, 525–549, 1984.

Jackson I. T., Downie P. A. — Abdominoplasty: the waistline stitch and other refinements. *Plast. Reconstr. Surg.*, *61*, 2, 180–3, 1978.

Jamra F. A. — Reconstruction of the umbilicus by a double VY procedure. *Plast. Reconstr. Surg.*, *64*, 1, 106–107, 1979.

Juri J., Juri C., Raiden G. — Reconstruction of the umbilicus in abdominoplasty. *Plast. Reconstr. Surg.*, *63*, 4, 580–582, 1979.

Kamper M. J., Dwight V., Galloway D. V., Aschley F. — Abdominal panniculectomy after massive weight loss. *Plast. Reconstr. Surg.*, *50*, 441–446, 1972.

Kanter M. A. — The lymphatic system: a historical perspective. *Plast. Reconstr. Surg.*, *79*, 1, 131–139, 1987.

Kelly H. A. — Report of gynecological cases: Case 3, excessive growth of fat. *Bull. John Hopkins Hosp.*, *10*, 197, 1899.

Kelly H. A. — Excision of the fat of the abdominal wall lipectomy. *Surg. Gynecol. Obstet.*, *10*, 229–231, 1910.

Kesselring U. K., Meyer R. — A suction curette for removal of excessive local deposits of subcutaneous fat. *Plast. Reconstr. Surg.*, *62*, 305, 1978.

Kirianoff T. G. — Making a new umbilicus when none exists. Case report. *Plast. Reconstr. Surg.*, *61*, 4, 603–604, 1978.

Knittle J. L. — Nombre et tailles des cellules adipeuses du sujet obèse. *Triangle*, *13*, 2, 57–62, 1974.

Lagache G., Vandenbussche F. — Indication, contre-indications et résultats de la technique de Callia dans le traitement des ptoses cutanées abdominales avec ou sans surcharge graisseuse. *Ann. Chir. Plast.*, *16*, 1, 37–50, 1971.

Lagrot F. — A propos des dermolipectomies abdominales. *Bordeaux Chir.*, *3*, 221, 1970.

Le Kieffre M. — Chirurgie esthétique de l'abdomen. *Gaz. Méd. France*, *75*, 5605–5610, 1968.

Marchac D., Weston J. — Abdominoplasty in infants for removal of giant congenital nevi: a report of 3 cases. *Plast. Reconstr. Surg.*, *75*, 2, 155–158, 1985.

Marchal G., Lapeyrie H., Amar E. — Sur un procédé de plastie cutanée dans le traitement des faiblesses et du tablier adipeux de la paroi abdominale. *Montpellier Chir.*, *10*, 4, 315, 1964.

Mitz V., Elbaz J. S., Vilde F. — Etude des fibres élastiques dermiques au cours d'opérations plastiques du tronc. *Ann. Chir. Plast.*, *1*, 31–44, 1975.

Morel-Lavallée. — Epanchements traumatiques de sérosités. *Mémoires Originaux de l'Académie de Chirurgie*, 691–731, 1853.

Paturet G. — *Anatomie humaine*, tome III, fasc. I. Masson, Paris, 1951.

Picaud A. J., Sabatier P. H. – D'une technique de lipectomie qui garde ses indications précises. *XXIIIᵉ Congrès National de la Société Italienne de Chirurgie Plastique*, Turin, 1973.

Pierard J., Kint A., Barsaques J. De — *L'élastose sénile. Maladies du tissu élastique cutané*, pp. 373–388. Masson, Paris, 1968.

Pierard J., Barsaques J. De, Kint A. — *Le tissu élastique cutané normal. Maladie due tissu élastique cutané*, pp. 1–58, Masson, Paris, 1968.

Pitanguy I. — Abdominal lipectomy: an approach to it through an analysis of 300 consecutive cases. *Plastic. Reconstr. Surg.*, *40*, 4, 384–391, 1967.

Pitanguy I. — *Aesthetic plastic surgery of head and body*. Springer, Berlin, 1981.

Pitanguy I., Ceravolo M. P. — Our experience with combined procedures in aesthetic plastic surgery. *Plast. Reconstr. Surg.*, *71*, 56–63, 1983.

Planas J. — The « vest over pants » abdominoplasty. *Plast. Reconstr. Surg.*, *61*, 5, 694–700, 1978.

Pompeo De Pina D. — Aesthetic abdominal deformities: A personal approach to the posterior rectus sheath and rectus muscles. *Plast. Reconstr. Surg.*, *75*, 5, 660–667, 1985.

Pratt J. H., Irons G. B. — Panniculectomy and abdominoplasty. *Am. J. Obstet. Gynecol.*, *132*, 2, 165–168, 1978.

Psillakis J. M. — Plastic surgery of the abdomen with improvement in the body contour. Physiopathology and treatment of the aponeurotic musculature. *Clin. Plast. Surg.*, *11*, 3, 465–477, 1984.

Quenu J. — *Opérations sur les parois de l'abdomen et sur le tube digestif*. Masson, Paris, 1967.

Rebello C., Franco T. — Abdominoplasty through a sub-mammary incision. *Int. J. Surg.*, *62*, 9, 462–463, 1977.

Regnault P. — Abdominoplasty by the W-technique. *Plast. Reconstr. Surg.*, *55*, 272–275, 1965.

Rene L. — La laparoplastie. *Gaz. Méd. France*, 60, 22, 1247, 1953.

Richer P. — *Nouvelle anatomie artistique du corps humain.* Plon-Nourrit et Cie, Paris, 1906.

Ricketts R. R. — Simultaneous umbilicoplasty and closure of small omphaloceles. *Surg. Gynecol. Obstet.*, 157, 8, 572-573, 1983.

Robert B., Robert L. — Aging of connective tissues. General considerations. *In: Frontiers of matrix biology.* Karger, Bâle, 1973.

Robert B., Robert L. — Le vieillissement du conjonctif. *Triangle*, 14, 2, 163-171, 1974.

Robert L. — Rapport sur le symposium européen du tissu conjonctif de Padoue. *Concours Méd.*, suppl. n° 4, 8-13, 1974.

Robert L. — Le tissu conjonctif et la médecine moderne. *Concours Méd.*, suppl. n° 4, 3-5, 1975.

Robertson J. L. — Complications of « dermolipectomy » as an encore to abdominal operative procedure. *S. Afr. Med. J.*, 56, 4, 141-143, 1979.

Rouviére H. — *Anatomie des lymphatiques de l'homme.* Masson, Paris, 1981.

Rouviére H. — *Anatomie humaine descriptive et topographique*, tomes 2 et 3. Masson, Paris, 1984.

Ryan R. F. — Which patient needs the abdominoplasty? *Plast. Reconstr. Surg.*, 59, 6, 842-843, 1977.

Sabatier P. H., Barraya L., Picaud A. J. — Une technique originale de réfection de l'ombilic. *Ann. Chir. Plast.*, 23, 4, 245-248, 1978.

Salmon M. — *Artères de la peau: étude anatomique et chirurgicale.* Masson, Paris, 1936.

Sappey P. C. — *Anatomie, physiologie, pathologie des vaisseaux lymphatiques.* Adrien Delahaye, Paris, 1874.

Savage R. C. — Abdominoplasty following gastrointestinal bypass surgery. *Plast. Reconstr. Surg.*, 71, 4, 500-509, 1983.

Schepelmann E. — Ueber baucheenkenplastik mit besonderer Berücksichtigung des Hängebanches. *Beitr. Klin. Chir.*, 111, 372, 1918.

Schrudde J. — Lipexeresis or a means of eliminating local adiposity. *Aesth. Plast. Surg.*, 4, 215, 1980.

Schurte M., Letterman G. — A suggested English nomenclature for aesthetic surgery of the abdominal wall. *Aesthet. Plast. Surg.*, 6, 2, 99-100, 1982.

Schurter M., Letterman G. — Abdominoplasty or abdominal dermolipectomy. *Ann. Plast. Surg.*, 2, 3, 235-238, 1979.

Serson Neto D. — Abdominoplasty. *Aesthet. Plast. Surg.*, 6, 1, 1-5, 1982.

Serson Neto D. — Dermolipectomia abdominal: abordagem geometrica. *IXe Congresso Latino-Americano de Cirurgia Plastica*, Bogota (Colombia), 1969.

Sher W. et coll. — Repair of abdominal wall defects: gore-tex vs marlex graft. *Am. Surg.*, 46, 11, 618-623, 1980.

Simkoff A. A., Elbaz J. S. — L'hypotension contrôlée, une technique d'anesthésie injustement méconnue en chirurgie plastique. *Ann. Chir. Plast.*, 19, 4, 353-360, 1974.

Souza Pinto E. B. — A new methodology in abdominal aesthetic surgery. *Aesthet. Plast. Surg.*, 11, 213-222, 1987.

Stuckey J. G. — Midabdomen abdominoplasty. *Plast. Reconstr. Surg.*, 63, 3, 333-335, 1979.

Talaat S. M. et coll. — Inverted T incision in abdominoplasty and incisional hernias. *J. Egypt. Med. Assoc.*, 60, 7-8, 664-666, 1977.

Testut L. — *Anatomie Humaine*, tome II, p. 364. G. Doin. Paris, 1948.

Thomeret G. — La lipectomie circulaire. *Nouv. Pratique Chir. Illustrée*, 169, 1971.

Thorek M. — *Plastic surgery of the breast and abdominal wall.* Ch. C. Thomas, Springfield, 11, 1942.

Vandenbussche F., Meresse B., Debaere P. A., Vandevoorde J., Lagache G. — Indications morphologiques et choix de la technique opératoire dans les lipectomies. *Ve Congrès de l'IPRS*, 1975.

Vandenbussche F., Meresse B., Lagache G. — Chirurgie des excédents cutanéo-graisseux corporels; choix techniques en fonction du type de surcharge. *Riv. Ital. Chir. Plast.*, 5, 3-4, 369-395, 1973.

Vernon S. — Umbilical transplantation upward and abdominal contouring in lipectomy. *Am. J. Surg.*, 94, 490-492, 1957.

Vilain R. — La technique dite « en soleil couchant » dans les dermo-dystrophies abdominales. *Ann. Chir. Plast.*, 20, 2, 239-242, 1975.

Vilain R. — Traitement des stéatoméries chez la femme: théorie et pratique. *Ann. Chir. Plast.*, 20, 2, 135-146, 1975.

Vilain R. — A propos de la chirurgie réparatrice de la paroi abdominale. *Bull. Mens. Soc. Chir.* (Paris) 54, 290-294, 1964.

Vilain R. — Chirurgie raisonnable de l'obésité. *In: Chirurgie et Spécialités, Entretien de Bichat.* p. 161, Expansion Scientifique Française, Paris, 1958.

Vilain R., Dardour J. C., Bzowski A. — Use of dermal-fat flaps in treating abdominal scars, in abdominoplasty, and in subtrochanteric lipectomy. *Plast. Reconstr. Surg.*, 60, 6, 876-881, 1977.

Vilain R., Dubousset J. — Technique et indications de la lipectomie circulaire. *Ann. Chir.*, 18, 289-300, 1964.

Vilain R., Dardour J. C., Staub S., Mitz V. — Dix questions à propos de l'aspiration de la graisse par la technique d'Y.G. Illouz. *Ann. Chir. Plast. Esthét*, 29, 2, 180-184, 1984.

Vilain R., Elbaz J. S., Singlier P., Gueriot J., Clelirzin R. — Etude critique des complications des laparotomies. *Ann. Chir. Plast.*, 21, 5-6, 262-288, 1967.

Vilain R., Monsaingeon J. — Rapport du XIe colloque international de dermo-chirurgie sur le vieillissement de la peau. *Ann. Chir. Plast.*, 17, 1, 92-93, 1973.

Voloir P. — Opérations plastiques sus-aponévrotiques sur la paroi abdominale antérieure. *Thèse Méd.*, Paris, 1960.

Voss S., Shorp H., Scott J. — Abdominoplasty combined with gynecological surgical procedures. *Obstet. Gynecol.*, 67, 2, 181-185, 1986.

Wallace A. F. — Cosmetic surgery of the abdomen, eyelids, face and chin. *Practitioner*, 224, 1342, 414-419, 1980.

Walsh J. J., Bonnar J., Wright F. W. — A study of pulmonary embolism and deep leg vein thrombosis after major gynaecological surgery using labelled fibrinogen phlebography and lungs. *J. Obstet. Gynecol. Br. Comm.*, 81, 311-316, 1974.

Wilkinson T., Swartz B. — Individual modification in body contour surgery: the « limited » abdominoplasty. *Plast. Reconstr. Surg.*, 77, 5, 779-784, 1986.

Wlodarczyk B., Soussaline M. — Toward a more natural

umbilicus in abdominoplasty. *Ann. Chir. Plast. Esthét.*, 29, 1, 90–91, 1984.

Wood R. — Abdominoplasty: agony and ectasy. *Aesthet. Plast. Surg.*, 9, 1, 51–56, 1985.

Zumer L., Baux S., Mole B. — Les plasties abdominales à visée esthétiques: variantes techniques. *Ann. Chir. Plast. Esthét.*, 26, 4, 383–385, 1981.

Index